NATIONAL ACADEMIES *Sciences Engineering Medicine*

NATIONAL ACADEMIES PRESS
Washington, DC

Psychological Factors That Contribute to the Dearth of Black Students in Science, Engineering, and Medicine

Evelynn Hammonds,
Shirley Malcom, Vivian Pinn, and
Paula Whitacre, *Rapporteurs*

Cato T. Laurencin, *Editor*

Roundtable on Black Men and
Black Women in Science,
Engineering, and Medicine

Policy and Global Affairs

Health and Medicine Division

Proceedings of a Workshop

NATIONAL ACADEMIES PRESS 500 Fifth Street, NW Washington, DC 20001

This activity was supported by contracts between the National Academy of Sciences and Aetna Foundation (#18-8876), Johnson & Johnson, the National Institutes of Health (HHSN263201800029I/75N98021F00006), the National Research Council President's Circle Fund, the University of Pittsburgh, and the W. K. Kellogg Foundation. Any opinions, findings, conclusions, or recommendations expressed in this publication do not necessarily reflect the views of any organization or agency that provided support for the project.

International Standard Book Number: 978-0-309-69285-4
International Standard Book Number: 0-309-69285-7
Digital Object Identifier: https://doi.org/10.17226/26691

This publication is available from the National Academies Press, 500 Fifth Street, NW, Keck 360, Washington, DC 20001; (800) 624-6242 or (202) 334-3313; http://www.nap.edu.

Printed in the United States of America.

Suggested citation: National Academies of Sciences, Engineering, and Medicine. 2023. *Psychological Factors That Contribute to the Dearth of Black Students in Science, Engineering, and Medicine: Proceedings of a Workshop*. Washington, DC: The National Academies Press. https://doi.org/10.17226/26691.

The **National Academy of Sciences** was established in 1863 by an Act of Congress, signed by President Lincoln, as a private, nongovernmental institution to advise the nation on issues related to science and technology. Members are elected by their peers for outstanding contributions to research. Dr. Marcia McNutt is president.

The **National Academy of Engineering** was established in 1964 under the charter of the National Academy of Sciences to bring the practices of engineering to advising the nation. Members are elected by their peers for extraordinary contributions to engineering. Dr. John L. Anderson is president.

The **National Academy of Medicine** (formerly the Institute of Medicine) was established in 1970 under the charter of the National Academy of Sciences to advise the nation on medical and health issues. Members are elected by their peers for distinguished contributions to medicine and health. Dr. Victor J. Dzau is president.

The three Academies work together as the **National Academies of Sciences, Engineering, and Medicine** to provide independent, objective analysis and advice to the nation and conduct other activities to solve complex problems and inform public policy decisions. The National Academies also encourage education and research, recognize outstanding contributions to knowledge, and increase public understanding in matters of science, engineering, and medicine.

Learn more about the National Academies of Sciences, Engineering, and Medicine at **www.nationalacademies.org**.

Consensus Study Reports published by the National Academies of Sciences, Engineering, and Medicine document the evidence-based consensus on the study's statement of task by an authoring committee of experts. Reports typically include findings, conclusions, and recommendations based on information gathered by the committee and the committee's deliberations. Each report has been subjected to a rigorous and independent peer-review process and it represents the position of the National Academies on the statement of task.

Proceedings published by the National Academies of Sciences, Engineering, and Medicine chronicle the presentations and discussions at a workshop, symposium, or other event convened by the National Academies. The statements and opinions contained in proceedings are those of the participants and are not endorsed by other participants, the planning committee, or the National Academies.

Rapid Expert Consultations published by the National Academies of Sciences, Engineering, and Medicine are authored by subject-matter experts on narrowly focused topics that can be supported by a body of evidence. The discussions contained in rapid expert consultations are considered those of the authors and do not contain policy recommendations. Rapid expert consultations are reviewed by the institution before release.

For information about other products and activities of the National Academies, please visit www.nationalacademies.org/about/whatwedo.

PSYCHOLOGICAL FACTORS ACTION GROUP PLANNING COMMITTEE

EVELYNN M. HAMMONDS (*Co-Chair*), Harvard University
SHIRLEY M. MALCOM (*Co-Chair)*, American Association for the Advancement of Science
VIVIAN W. PINN (*Co-Chair*), NIH Fogarty International Center
KEVIN COKLEY, The University of Texas at Austin
MICHELLENE DAVIS, Esq., National Medical Fellowships, Inc.
GARTH N. GRAHAM, Aetna, Inc.
THOMAS VANCE, Boys & Girls Clubs of America

Project Staff

MARIA LUND DAHLBERG, Senior Program Officer, Roundtable on Black Men and Black Women in Science, Engineering, and Medicine
LYNNETTE LUSENAKA, Program Officer, Roundtable on Black Men and Black Women in Science, Engineering, and Medicine
REGINALD HAYES, Associate Program Officer, Roundtable on Black Men and Black Women in Science, Engineering, and Medicine
MARQUITA WHITING, Senior Program Assistant, Roundtable on Black Men and Black Women in Science, Engineering, and Medicine
TOM ARRISON, Program Director, Policy and Global Affairs (until May 2021)
PAULA WHITACRE, Consultant Writer

ROUNDTABLE ON BLACK MEN AND BLACK WOMEN IN SCIENCE, ENGINEERING, AND MEDICINE

CATO T. LAURENCIN (NAS/NAE/NAM) (*Chair*), University of Connecticut Health
OLUJIMI AJIJOLA, UCLA Medical Center
GILDA A. BARABINO (NAE/NAM), Olin College of Engineering
CHARLES R. BRIDGES, JR., Janssen Research & Development, LLC
CEDRIC BRIGHT, East Carolina University
L. D. BRITT (NAM), Eastern Virginia Medical School
ANDRÉ L. CHURCHWELL, Vanderbilt University School of Medicine
THEODORE CORBIN, Drexel University
GEORGE Q. DALEY (NAM), Harvard Medical School
WAYNE FREDERICK, Howard University
PAULA T. HAMMOND (NAS/NAE/NAM), Massachusetts Institute of Technology
EVELYNN M. HAMMONDS (NAM), Harvard University
LYNNE M. HOLDEN, Montefiore Medical Center
CAMARA P. JONES, Morehouse School of Medicine
CORA BAGLEY MARRETT, University of Wisconsin–Madison
VALERIE MONTGOMERY RICE (NAM), Morehouse School of Medicine
RANDALL C. MORGAN, JR., W. Montague Cobb/NMA Health Institute
ELIZABETH O. OFILI (NAM), Morehouse School of Medicine
VIVIAN W. PINN (NAM), National Institutes of Health (Retired)
JOAN Y. REEDE (NAM), Harvard Medical School
LOUIS W. SULLIVAN (NAM), Morehouse School of Medicine
HANNAH VALANTINE (NAM), Stanford University
CLYDE W. YANCY (NAM), Northwestern University
MARK ALEXANDER (Ex Officio Member), 100 Black Men of America, Inc.
MARIE BERNARD (Ex Officio Member), National Institutes of Health
KIMBERLY BRYANT (Ex Officio Member), Black Girls CODE
IVORY DEAN (Ex Officio Member), Chan Zuckerberg Initiative
GARTH N. GRAHAM (NAM) (Ex Officio Member), Google, Inc.
IAN HENRY (Ex Officio Member), Procter & Gamble Company

ORLANDO KIRTON (Ex Officio Member), Society of Black Academic Surgeons
JOHN R. LUMPKIN (NAM) (Ex Officio Member), Blue Cross and Blue Shield of North Carolina Foundation
SHIRLEY MALCOM (NAS) (Ex Officio Member), American Association for the Advancement of Science
ALFRED MAYS (Ex Officio Member), Burroughs Wellcome Fund
LAMONT R. TERRELL (Ex Officio Member), GlaxoSmithKline

Project Staff

MARIA LUND DAHLBERG, Senior Program Officer, Roundtable on Black Men and Black Women in Science, Engineering, and Medicine
ANDRÉ PORTER, Senior Program Officer, Roundtable on Black Men and Black Women in Science, Engineering, and Medicine (*from June 2022*)
LYNNETTE LUSENAKA, Program Officer, Roundtable on Black Men and Black Women in Science, Engineering, and Medicine (*until June 2022*)
REGINALD HAYES, Associate Program Officer, Roundtable on Black Men and Black Women in Science, Engineering, and Medicine
MARQUITA WHITING, Senior Program Assistant, Roundtable on Black Men and Black Women in Science, Engineering, and Medicine (*until September 2022*)
KARLA RILEY, Senior Program Assistant, Roundtable on Black Men and Black Women in Science, Engineering, and Medicine (*from September 2022*)
TOM ARRISON, Program Director, Policy and Global Affairs (*until May 2021*)
PAULA WHITACRE, Consultant Writer

Preface

It is an honor for me to serve as chair of the National Academies of Sciences, Engineering, and Medicine Roundtable on Black Men and Black Women in Science, Engineering, and Medicine, and serve as the editor of the first in a series of proceedings publications from the Roundtable. Our work began in 2015 when leaders of the W. Montague Cobb/National Medical Association Health Institute and I recognized the growing absence of Black men in medical schools. In fact, levels of Black men entering medical school reached a historic low in 2015 and 2016. Starting in 2016, and with financial support from important partners such as the Aetna Foundation, the Burroughs Wellcome Fund, the Robert Wood Johnson Foundation, and the Connecticut Black and Puerto Rican Legislative Caucus, we began planning a National Academies workshop on issues surrounding the absence of Black men in medicine. The joint workshop entitled "The Growing Absence of Black Men in Medicine and Science" took place in 2017. It was historic, in that to my knowledge it was the first National Academies activity specifically focused on issues involving Black people. The proceedings is entitled *An American Crisis: The Growing Absence of Black Men in Medicine and Science*. It was released in May 2018, and corresponded to a briefing on the subject of Black men and medicine with the Congressional Black Caucus in Washington, D.C. Many of the ideas that emerged from the workshop have been embraced by academia, industry, and philanthropy. More needs to be done.

Our next steps have involved the development of a more permanent presence in the National Academies to discuss issues surrounding Black men and Black women in science, engineering, and medicine. With support from our anchor partners named above, along with the Johnson & Johnson Company, the W. K. Kellogg Foundation, and the University of Pittsburg, and with the continued leadership and commitment from Dr. Victor Dzau, the president of the National Academy of Medicine, the Roundtable on Black Men and Black Women in Science, Engineering, and Medicine was launched late in 2018. I am grateful to the steering committee members for the Roundtable: Drs. L. D. Britt, Cedric M. Bright, George Q. Daley, Randall C. Morgan Jr., Elizabeth O. Ofili, Vivian W. Pinn, and Louis W. Sullivan.

In September 2021, the Roundtable organized a workshop aimed at exploring psychological factors that contribute to the dearth of Black students in science, engineering, and medicine. From the outset, the goal of the workshop was to gather ideas that might address the systemic and long-term changes needed to allow for success of Black students. The co-chairs for this workshop spent considerable time examining the continuum of systemic issues that affect Black students. The workshop began with discussing Pre-K to 12 education as a fundamental issue for Black students. How does one address foundational effects of a system often broken? Next, a discussion of changes needed at colleges and universities took place. The question was asked: How does one not only assure access and success but also promote well-being? Next, a discussion of other sectors that can influence outcomes was discussed, and finally, an ideas session took place, noting a sense of urgency in moving forward with change. The overall goal of the workshop was to explore innovative ideas that could ultimately become policies to help ensure the success and vitality of Blacks pursuing careers in science, engineering, and medicine in a world fraught with systemic pressures.

I am grateful to the co-chairs of the workshop, Dr. Evelynn M. Hammonds, Dr. Shirley M. Malcom, and Dr. Vivian W. Pinn. This was perhaps the most difficult and controversial subject that the Roundtable has tackled so far. They demonstrated a high level of intellectual expertise combined with a sense of compassion and urgency to the workshop program. This workshop provided a 360-degree view of issues surrounding psychological barriers for Blacks pursuing science, engineering, and medicine. I look forward to seeing follow-on discussions on how the ideas here can be implemented in partnership with multiple sectors, especially education. As with the Roundtable's previous proceedings, they are meant to move us to action.

Cato T. Laurencin, M.D., Ph.D. (NAS/NAE/NAM)
Chair, Roundtable on Black Men and Black Women
in Science, Engineering, and Medicine
University Professor, University of Connecticut

Acknowledgments

This Proceedings of a Workshop was prepared by the workshop rapporteurs as a factual summary of what was presented and discussed at the workshop. The planning committee's role was limited to planning and convening the workshop. The statements made are those of the rapporteurs and do not necessarily represent positions of the workshop participants as a whole, the planning committee, or the National Academies of Sciences, Engineering, and Medicine. We wish to extend sincere thanks to all the members of the planning committee for their contributions in scoping, developing, and carrying out this project.

This Proceedings of a Workshop was reviewed in draft form by individuals chosen for their diverse perspectives and technical expertise. The purpose of this independent review is to provide candid and critical comments that will assist the National Academies of Sciences, Engineering, and Medicine in making each published proceedings as sound as possible and to ensure that it meets the institutional standards for quality, objectivity, evidence, and responsiveness to the charge. The review comments and draft manuscript remain confidential to protect the integrity of the process. We wish to thank the following individuals for their review of these proceedings: George Daley, Harvard University; Keivan Stassun, Vanderbilt University; and Clyde Yancy, Northwestern University. Although the reviewers listed above provided many constructive comments and suggestions, they were not asked to endorse the content of the proceedings, nor did they see the final draft before its release. The review of this proceedings was overseen by Cora Marrett, University of Wisconsin–Madison (ret.). Appointed by the National Academies, she was responsible for making certain that an independent examination of this report was carried out in accordance with the standards of the National Academies and that all review comments were carefully considered. Responsibility for the final content rests entirely with the rapporteurs and the National Academies.

Contents

1

Introduction

Efforts over the last several decades to increase the participation and leadership of Black men and women in the nation's scientific and medical workforce have had limited results. Despite many individual successes, the number of Black professionals in science, engineering, and medicine (SEM) fields has not reached a level that corresponds with African American representation in the country at large. Structural racism affects progress at all stages along the pathway—from young children through graduate and medical students through faculty and clinicians at all levels. Beyond entry into educational programs or recruitment into workplaces seeking to diversify, challenges persist to achieve equity and inclusion for Black males and females. Moreover, psychological barriers confound the engagement of Black men and women in SEM fields.

To explore these issues and suggest solutions, the National Academies of Sciences, Engineering, and Medicine (the National Academies) launched the Roundtable on Black Men and Black Women in Science, Engineering, and Medicine. Over the past 2 years, the Roundtable has convened workshops on K–12 education, the impact of COVID-19, financial burdens to pursuing SEM careers, and other topics. Sessions during each of these workshops identified psychological factors related to those specific topics. To have a more targeted discussion, the Roundtable convened a virtual workshop on September 14–15, 2021, entitled "Psychological Factors that Contribute to the Dearth of Black Students in Science, Engineering, and Medicine." As summarized in this proceedings, panelists and participants identified policies and practices that perpetuate these factors and explored solutions toward achieving and maintaining wellness, especially among students and young professionals.

OPENING REMARKS

Welcome from the National Academies Leadership

Laura Castillo-Page, Ph.D. (the National Academies) welcomed participants and shared her priorities as the National Academies inaugural chief diversity and inclusion officer. "Although DEI [diversity, equity, and inclusion] work is not new to the National Academies, I am establishing a new office that will be a resource for the entire organization," Dr. Castillo-Page explained. "As many of you know, this requires a comprehensive and cross-cutting approach where we can successfully address the cultural and systemic changes that are necessary to advance equity, diversity, inclusion, and antiracism within our organization." The office's priorities include building the National Academies' capacity to advance diversity, equity, and inclusion internally and in outwardly facing work. Internal priorities include improving the workplace culture for staff, members, and volunteers. External priorities relate to workshops and consensus studies across the National Academies' seven programmatic areas.

"This is why I am so pleased to see the many accomplishments of the Roundtable even before others were prepared to discuss these issues, let alone take action against them," she said. "The work of the Roundtable is a model for the Academies on how to unpack, understand, and generate solutions for advancing Black men and Black women in science, engineering, and medicine."

Dr. Castillo-Page noted the importance of the workshop focus because mental health and psychological factors not only impact access to careers but also impact communities of color more generally. She noted in her own background growing up in Harlem, she saw firsthand how these factors affected her family and community.

Background on the Roundtable

Roundtable chair Cato Laurencin, M.D., Ph.D. (University of Connecticut), thanked Roundtable members, National Academies staff, and participants. He noted his own recent book draws on many of the issues that the Roundtable addresses (Laurencin, forthcoming).

As Dr. Laurencin explained, the origins of the Roundtable began with a 2018 workshop and subsequent publication about the crisis resulting from the growing absence of Black men in medicine (NASEM, 2018). Articles in the media were asking whether Black males in medicine were becoming an "endangered species," he recounted. There has been a rebound in numbers, he noted, but much work remains.

After a meeting with members of the Congressional Black Caucus to discuss the workshop, the National Academies established the Roundtable on Black Men and Black Women in Science, Engineering, and Medicine in 2019, and Dr. Laurencin expressed his appreciation to Roundtable members and sponsors. As he elaborated, the goal of the Roundtable is to understand issues and create ideas for solutions, especially solutions utilizing the strengths in having Black men and Black women in these fields. At its inaugural meeting in December 2019, the group decided that each subsequent meeting would include data gathering, ideas generation, and a public workshop. Action groups were formed to foster information sharing and development of evidence-based approaches, engage with stakeholders, and conduct a range of activities for meaningful change. Seven action groups have been established: public engagement; mentorship and advising; systemic change to overcome psychological barriers to success; racism; pre-K to graduate education; financing; and COVID-19. With the current workshop, each action group has organized at least one workshop, and proceedings have been published (NASEM 2020, 2021, 2022 a, b, c)

In reviewing the workshop's Statement of Task (see Box 1-1) and agenda (see Appendix A), Dr. Laurencin stressed the need to move beyond incremental interventions to create large and systemic changes. "This is a workshop and not a talk-shop," he stressed. "We have to move forward with urgency."

Context of the Workshop

Workshop co-chair Vivian Pinn, M.D. (National Institutes of Health), spoke on behalf of herself; fellow co-chairs Shirley Malcom, Ph.D. (American Association for the Advancement of Science [AAAS]); and Evelynn Hammonds, Ph.D. (Harvard University); and the planning committee. Dr. Pinn shared the mission statement of the Mental Health and Behavioral Action Group used as the basis to plan the workshop:

> This action group will examine the mental health, psychological, and behavioral factors that contribute to the dearth of Black men

BOX 1-1
Workshop Statement of Task

This workshop will examine the psychological factors that contribute to the persistent dearth of Black students in science, engineering, and medicine (SEM). Workshop speakers and participants will identify policies and practices that perpetuate those factors and lay a foundation of knowledge for others to more effectively engage on these issues. The workshop discussion will focus on systemic solutions to address the major impediments to access and success for Black students and scholars in SEM. Major objectives of the workshop include:

(1) examining psychological barriers that contribute to decreased representation of Black students in SEM, including the chronic environmental stressors that contribute to anxiety, depression, and substance use and abuse as well as the racially insensitive educational barriers that Black youth face; (2) exploring solutions to overcoming negative stereotypes and systemic racism and biases that prevent Black students from pursuing careers in SEM; (3) assisting stakeholders in moving beyond incremental interventions toward more systemic changes, including policy changes that can support Black students, scientists, engineers, and physicians, and in turn strengthen their academic and racial identity and enhance their mental health.

> and Black women in American medicine and careers in science, engineering, and medicine and the dialectical tensions of risk and resilience. In the face of systemic racism, racialized sexism, discrimination, and racial microaggressions, Black youth face unique educational barriers that dehumanize them, undermine their academic confidence and motivation, weaken their academic self-concept, and perpetuate feelings of the imposter syndrome and stereotype threat reactions.

The committee looked at the work of the other Roundtable action groups to explore how mental health relates to each of them. "That allowed us to pull together all of the activities across the Roundtable in a comprehensive manner," she observed. For example, she said, the research literature shows that Black youth are disproportionately punished, suspended, and expelled in schools and are especially susceptible to the form of bias known as *adultification*, in which Black girls are hypersexualized and viewed as less innocent, and Black boys are viewed as older, less innocent, and more guilty of crimes. "These psychological factors and racial biases contribute to the theme of risk as the dominant narrative surrounding Black youth," she said, and called for a counternarrative of resilience to focus on strengths and factors related to success rather than failure. "We hear the negatives about our Black youth; we want to focus on the positives and the factors that contribute to success," she stressed.

She emphasized the need to focus on strategies and actions. "Yes, we need more research—but there is a lot that is known. We want to move from discussion to action," she said. "Also, we are focusing on systemic changes? Why is there always a focus on changing our Black youth to fit the system? Why are we not looking at what the system needs to do to better accommodate our Black youth?"

ORGANIZATION OF THIS PROCEEDINGS

The remainder of this publication is organized to follow the agenda of the workshop. Chapter 2 addresses mental health and socio-psychological factors to increase the participation of Black men and women in science, engineering, and medicine, including a keynote address by Altha Stewart, M.D., the first Black president of the American Psychiatric Association. Chapter 3 focuses on early education as the pathway to success and includes a presentation by Edmund Gordon, Ph.D., a pioneer in the creation of Head Start and other early childhood programs. Chapter 4 looks at changes in colleges and universities, with four innovative programs highlighted. Chapters 5 and 6 address approaches in other public and private institutions, including government agencies, health-care organizations, and foundations. Young professionals share their own experiences in Chapter 7, followed by conversation among the planning committee members and with participants in Chapter 8. A closing keynote by Cora Marrett, Ph.D. (University of Wisconsin–Madison) pulls together some of the workshop themes. The agenda and biographical sketches of the speakers can be found in Appendixes A and B.

In accordance with the policies of the National Academies, workshop participants did not attempt to establish any conclusions or recommendations about needs and future directions, focusing instead on issues discussed by the speakers and workshop participants. In addition, the planning committee's role was limited to planning the workshop. This proceedings was prepared by the rapporteurs as a factual summary of what occurred at the workshop.

REFERENCES

Laurencin, C. 2021. *Success Is What You Leave Behind: Fostering Leadership and Innovation.* London, UK: Academic Press.

NASEM (National Academies of Sciences, Engineering, and Medicine). 2018. *An American Crisis: The Growing Absence of Black Men in Medicine and Science: Proceedings of a Joint Workshop.* Washington, DC: The National Academies Press. https://www.nap.edu/catalog/25130/an-american-crisis-the-growing-absence-of-black-men-in.

NASEM. 2020. *The Impacts of Racism and Bias on Black People Pursuing Careers in Science, Engineering, and Medicine.* Washington, DC: The National Academies Press. https://www.nap.edu/catalog/25849/the-impacts-of-racism-and-bias-on-black-people-pursuing-careers-in-science-engineering-and-medicine.

NASEM. 2021. *COVID-19 and the Present and Future of Black Communities: The Role of Black Physicians, Engineers, and Scientists.* Washington, DC: The National Academies Press. https://doi.org/10.17226/26146.

NASEM. 2022a. *Educational Pathways for Black Students in Science, Engineering, and Medicine: Exploring Barriers and Possible Interventions: Proceedings of a Workshop.* Washington, DC: The National Academies Press. https://doi.org/10.17226/26391.

NASEM. 2022b. *Understanding and Offsetting Financial Barriers for Black Students in Science, Engineering, and Medicine: Programs, Partnerships, and Pathways: Proceedings of a Workshop.* Washington, DC: The National Academies Press. https://doi.org/10.17226/26576.

NASEM. 2022c. *Mentoring of Black Graduate and Medical Students, Postdoctoral Scholars, and Early-Career Faculty in Science, Engineering, and Medicine: Proceedings of a Workshop.* Washington, DC: The National Academies Press. https://doi.org/10.17226/26462.

2

Addressing Mental Health and Socio-Psychological Factors to Increase the Participation of Black Women and Men in SEM

Highlights from the Presentations

- Science identity starts early and can be nurtured by family, community, educators, and SEM professionals so that young people can build on their own cultural wealth (Dr. Stewart).
- When students face adverse environmental conditions and other challenges, they need more than advice to "buck up." They need help to identify issues; get help if they need it; and not feel afraid, ashamed, or stigmatized (Dr. Stewart).
- Blacks are the most studied population of students but usually with a focus on problems or deficits, rather than intellectual strengths and achievements (Dr. Cokley).
- The imposter syndrome can particularly harm Black students who, in addition to the self-doubt felt by other students, are the targets of implicit or explicit bias (Dr. Cokley).
- Student debt, low stipends, inadequate health insurance, and other financial stressors are taking a toll on the physical and mental health of Black graduate students, including those who are high achieving and assumed to be financially stable (Dr. McGee).
- Asking students to be in charge of the care of their own selves when structural problems are impeding them is a disservice to their health and well-being (Dr. McGee).

In the first session, Altha Stewart, M.D. (University of Tennessee Health Science Center), set the stage for the workshop by discussing the psychological challenges that can impede progress by Black men and women in science, engineering, and medicine (SEM) careers, as well as the ways to protect young people from being adversely affected by these challenges. Planning committee member Kevin Cokley, Ph.D. (University of Texas at Austin), discussed Black intellectual achievement and the myths that disparage such achievement. Ebony O. McGee, Ph.D. (Peabody College), presented her research on the impact of financial stressors on the mental health of high-achieving Black graduate students. Planning committee member Thomas Vance, Ph.D. (The New School), served as respondent.

OPENING KEYNOTE: FOCUSING ON STRENGTHS, OVERCOMING "ACES"

As a Black woman and a practicing psychiatrist for more than 40 years, Dr. Stewart shared how she draws on her life experience and professional knowledge in the search for solutions to support the careers of Black men and women. She reminded the group, as a point of reference, that Black women make up only 2 percent of all science, technology, engineering, and mathematics (STEM) professionals, and more than 500,000 low-income and minority high school students are missing from Advanced Placement math and science courses. The percentage of Black physicians, according to the American Association of Medical Colleges, has remained at 5 percent, essentially unchanged since 1940.

Dr. Stewart highlighted psychological barriers that contribute to this underrepresentation, amplifying several points made by Dr. Vivian Pinn in her introduction (see Chapter 1). Early childhood experiences and environments are critical, she noted. "The adultification of Black youth disrupts normal child development that is the clear pathway to successful outcomes career-wise," Dr. Stewart stated. Chronic environmental stressors, which she termed *adverse childhood experiences* (ACEs), contribute to the development of anxiety, depression, and substance use. For many Black young people aspiring to careers, she cautioned, "the ACEs get in the way," starting as early as kindergarten. Educational barriers, including lack of academic opportunities and strict disciplinary processes that are different for Blacks than for white counterparts, can result in different outcomes, lower graduation rates, and less likelihood to go on to higher education, she added.

Racialized microaggressions, sexism, and discrimination can weaken academic self-concept, especially in the developmental years, she continued, pointing to the constant devaluing of what would otherwise be cultural capital. For example, a student hearing that "you will never excel" leads to a belief that the pursuit is not worth trying. "In a society and medical culture that is so deeply rooted in systemic racism and structural barriers that are based on race, the [low] number of Black doctors should come as no surprise," she asserted. Workshops such as this, she contended, are compelling the profession to take a hard look at strategies and solutions that will prove effective in improving the numbers.

According to Dr. Stewart, a SEM identity begins very early in life, showing up as small seeds of interest. "It is up to us to grow and nurture them [Black children] and to stay with them throughout the long journey once they begin on this path," she urged. "We know this is not an easy journey. Programs are deeply rooted in systems in which white supremacy and racism contribute to the creation of very oppressive environments that are experienced by all students of color, and certainly in different ways by Black students." She asked more experienced Black professionals to remember the support they received along their pathways to success and provide similar support to young people.

Dr. Stewart related that her own journey began as a candy striper volunteer at St. Jude's Hospital in Memphis, where she became comfortable around science and scientists. A high school science teacher expanded her thinking that she could not only work in a lab, but run one. Although she faced "bumps" from people who thought she should not aspire to be a doctor, she recounted, a health careers summer program at Harvard University was pivotal to her future. She particularly credits meeting psychiatrist Alvin Poussaint, M.D., who challenged her to not be stopped by obstacles along the way. Her family and community also provided critical protective factors, especially unconditional love and support, that allowed her to achieve her goals without falling prey to ACEs, she added.

Growing up in Memphis in the late 1950s, Dr. Stewart attended a previously all-male Catholic high school. Another teacher suggested she not set her career goals too high. "He said he did not want me to get hurt, but, in other words, he was stealing my cultural wealth," she asserted. "It's that cultural wealth that allows students to feel positive about their abilities to succeed." Racism cannot be denied, but what we have to do is provide support both on the content and skills development side and on the emotional psychological support side. Mentors must become enmeshed in overall support for their mentees. "I see medical students all the time who are the first generation to go to college who have such high hopes but also heavy burdens to be a success. They are literally killing themselves to achieve. We have to be the protective factors for this cohort of young people who we want to recruit, retain, and be successful as our colleagues in the field."

This, Dr. Stewart noted, is what Dr. Poussaint did for her. She urged the creation of STEM programs that take into consideration things that students do not openly share, such as the ACEs in their lives, pressures from home, and the micro- and macroaggressions they experience every day. "Let's remember we have to talk about those things," she said. "They cannot be single-dose interventions if we are going to help students learn to use their cultural wealth. We have all heard about grit as this thing that we just barrel and push through, but it comes at a great psychological cost. I can tell you with certainty that we cannot continue to inspire our young people to 'have grit' without understanding the cost."

She noted that both targeted and systemic solutions are needed to help students in today's fast-paced environment. "When students are in challenging situations, our job is not just to tell them to buck up," Dr. Stewart said. "Our job is to help them identify issues, get help if they need it, and not feel afraid, ashamed, or stigmatized. This allows students to have self-efficacy, self-confidence, and autonomy in thought."

IMPORTANCE OF THE MISSION: SETTING THE STAGE FOR CHANGE

The Interplay of Psychological and Environmental Factors for Black Students

Dr. Cokley discussed promoting resilience as critical to increasing the participation of Black youth in SEM. He began by underscoring that psychological factors cannot be divorced from the environment in which people live. "The onus is placed on the youth themselves without considering the environmental factors that impinge upon them," he commented. His presentation touched on the myth of Black anti-intellectualism, environmental risks, being a Black student in a SEM major, racial identity and SEM achievement, the imposter syndrome and stereotype threat, and Black student resilience in SEM.

Dr. Cokley noted that it is often asked why capable Black students fail to perform as well as white and Asian students. He said the reasons offered relate to preparation, ability, genes, motivation, peer culture, and psycho-social factors. "The dominant narrative surrounding Black students is characterized by deficit thinking," he said. "Deficit thinking focuses on presumed reactive racial identity that is believed to negatively impact achievement. No other group of students has been more studied or written about, but more misunderstood or more maligned."

Research paints a different picture, Dr. Cokley countered. For example, his own research affirms that Black students are intellectual, inquisitive, and engaged (Cokley, 2015). Culturally competent teachers can bring out students' best achievement, he said, which points to the importance of representation. Environmental risks that make full STEM participation difficult include systemic racism, racialized sexism, discrimination, and racial microaggressions, he added (Cokley, 2016). He also highlighted research on challenges related to being Black in STEM majors. For example, Basile and Black (2019) showed how Black students who try to join study groups or attend instructor office hours are frequently met with hostility and the message they do not belong. Dr. Cokley quoted a first-generation Black engineering student who said he received support from Black faculty and students elsewhere on campus, but none from his own department (McCoy et al., 2017). Dr. Cokley added, "This is indicative of the messages that Black students in STEM majors often receive."

Dr. Cokley's research has shown that "racial identity can be both a risk and a resilience factor in STEM achievement." It becomes a risk factor when students internalize miseducated stereotypes and "start to believe the negative chatter," he explained. In contrast, a racial identity that embraces being Black, has strong Black consciousness and awareness of history, and is aware of the reality of racism can serve as a positive factor. "I am not suggesting that a person has to primarily define themselves by their racial identity," he clarified. "What I am suggesting is that having a negative identity is bad for academic achievement." He noted Basile and Black (2019) identified three forms of racialization: (1) receiving messages that racial identity is only valued on paper, such as in recruitment; (2) receiving open or coded messages that Black students do not belong in SEM spaces; and (3) receiving messages of being considered special and unique because of race but also expected to assimilate to white ideals.

In recent years, Dr. Cokley reported, imposter phenomenon or syndrome has been identified as "the experience among academically or professionally successful individuals of feeling like a fraud." However, he observed the literature was not addressing the experience of Black students, and he began to look at the imposter phenomenon through a more culturally appropriate lens. Many Black students are trying to obtain a degree in the context of racially hostile campuses, marginalization, and discrimination from peers and faculty. He termed their questioning whether they belong as a racialized form of the imposter phenomenon that is separate from more general self-doubt that other students may face. The threat of being viewed through the lens of a negative stereotype can also lead to disidentification with school and pursuit of SEM majors, Dr. Cokley said, and these socio-psychological factors are linked to anxiety and depression.

"Black, Brilliant, and Broke": Graduate School, Semi-Poverty, and the Mental Health Crisis in SEM

Dr. McGee explained that her research focuses on the impact of financial and other structural issues on Black graduate students to feel authentic and whole in their work. She noted that many of her findings apply to undergraduate students.

Student debt is an important contributor to financial stress, Dr. McGee pointed out. Ninety percent of Black undergraduates take out student loans, compared with 66 percent of white students. Graduate loans have grown by $2.3 billion annually, and graduate-level loan fees and interest rates are higher than those for undergraduates. These factors widen the financial disparities between Black and white graduate students, she noted. Forty-four percent of graduating Black students, compared with 22 percent of white students, leave graduate school with debt. And in general, STEM students have more debt than non-STEM counterparts.

Graduate students often face the low wages, unsafe conditions, long hours, and lack of appreciation that have been characterized as conditions in fast food or warehouse positions, Dr. McGee commented. "Academia relies heavily on underpaid labor, increased enrollment, and merit-based scholarship," she said. "This 'corporatizing' of academia has had the most negative impact on scholars of color" (see Figure 2-1). Many choose to join the workforce with a B.S. degree because "they cannot be broke for 6 to 10 years as they earn graduate degrees," she commented.

Further disaggregating the data, women owe about $1 trillion of the nation's overall $1.7 trillion in student debt, Dr. McGee reported. Among all demographics, Black women have the highest rate of graduate student loan debt at an average of $75,085. Some women, she noted, are literally dying in their 60s and 70s with student debt. According to the National

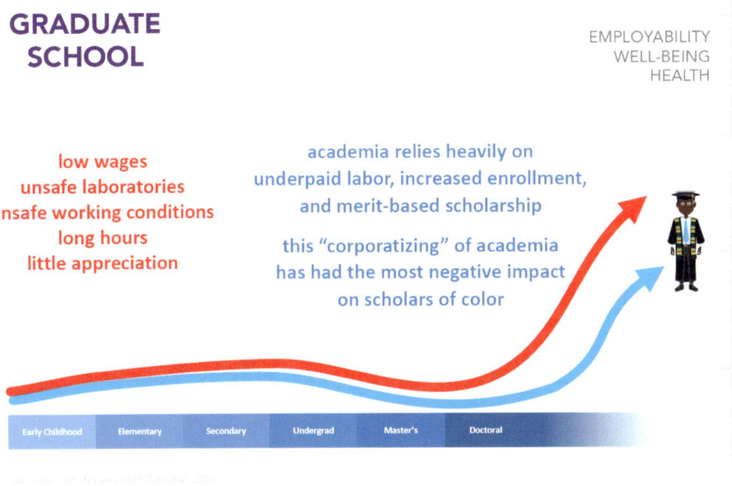

FIGURE 2-1 Low wages, long hours, and other common conditions in academia significantly harm scholars of color.
SOURCE: Ebony McGee, Workshop Presentation, September 14, 2021.

Science Foundation, she pointed out, women with the highest degrees in their fields earn about $30,000 less per year than their male counterparts.

Dr. McGee connected financial data with physical and emotional health. As context, she painted a picture of what students endure. "The culture needs to be interrogated," she asserted. "We have to say plainly that many fields in STEM were born out of eugenics. They were born out of warfare and economic domination.... We cannot separate ourselves from this culture. We cannot erase that narrative; the residue stays with us." Dr. McGee has researched situations that foment microaggressions, imposter syndrome, and toxic relationships for many years. Significantly, she continued, the impact of financial difficulties on health was not part of her initial research. "I, too, believed that the financial difficulties of a high-achieving STEM person were diminished," she commented. "But people are *not* okay. There is a silent, undertold agony of Black high achievers, with young scientists experiencing such conditions as anxiety attacks, self-medication, exhaustion, and miscarriages, among other conditions."

Her research is now trying to pull out these tensions. For example, her interview protocol now includes asking questions about how students are eating. She has heard from many Black female STEM graduate students who go on dates in hopes of a free meal, Black male STEM graduate students working in soup kitchens to eat, and other indications of food insecurity. In expanding her interview questions, she also found many students are sending home some of the little money they do earn, giving them fewer resources to live on. Black and Brown graduate students report they are often asked to babysit not only their relatives but also the children of their friends, neighbors, and even colleagues and faculty members.

She also started to ask students about health insurance. For many, health care is limited at best, with few culturally affirming medical professionals and limited mental health coverage available. Most insurance covers only a handful of sessions with a mental health provider, after which students must pay out of pocket. In any event, with few Black professionals in practice, "How do you talk to a white male psychiatrist about the racism experienced from your white male professor?" she asked rhetorically. "That is a set-up. Do they know about racial battle fatigue or minority stress? What kind of training and background do they have?"

She also referred to "the myth of me-me-me self-care," such as massages or expensive coffee drinks, as a flawed option for wellness. "I am arguing that asking students to be in charge of the care of their own selves when structural problems are impeding them is a disservice to self-care," she stated. She noted that universities and the governments that receive tax dollars from Black STEM students have a responsibility to provide essential services.

To change the landscape of STEM, Dr. McGee called not only for more representation at the table but also to include structural equity at the table. Policies and practices could include antiracist institutional health policies and practices; reparations for Black STEM professionals in the form of venture capital for STEM entrepreneurship; redistribution of STEM wealth creation; dismantling of the insurance industry; and culturally affirming reconstruction of Eurocentric STEM disciplines, she suggested. Dr. McGee concluded by sharing two resources that she developed: the Explorations in Diversifying Engineering Faculty Initiative and the Institute in Critical Quantitative and Mixed Methodologies Training for Underrepresented Scholars.[1]

---

[1] For information about these resources, see https://www.teamedefi.org and https://www.icqcm.org, respectively.

DISCUSSION

When Dr. Vance further questioned Dr. McGee about her ideas to achieve structural equity and inclusion in a given institution, she acknowledged the difficulty but urged not shying away from the work. It may mean bringing in outside consultants rather than tasking Black and Brown faculty with fixing the system and putting themselves on the line, she suggested. A participant who identified herself as an Asian American woman asked what allies can do to help fix the system. Dr. McGee noted it depends on each situation's micro culture and politics, as well as an individual's position and level of power. Generally, she suggested that there is strength in people coming together on shared issues of being oppressed.

To close the session, Dr. Cokley returned to his earlier points. "Black students are under the most scrutiny of any group of students," he said. "We must help them navigate racist environments. Part of what I struggle with as a psychologist is that we have only so much control over our lives. You take the brightest and most capable students and place them in hostile, toxic environments, and it becomes a miracle they can even make it out! It is a 'both/and situation' to help them navigate the environment and not internalize toxic messages, while also prepare and inoculate them to become resilient."

REFERENCES

Basile, V., and R. Black. 2019. They hated me till I was one of the "good ones": Toward understanding and disrupting the differential racialization of undergraduate African American STEM majors. *The Journal of Negro Education* 88(3): 379–390.

Cokley, K. O. 2015. *The Myth of Black Anti-Intellectualism: A True Psychology of African American Students*. Santa Barbara, CA: Praeger.

Cokley, K. O. 2016. What it means to be black in the American educational system. *The Conversation*. https://theconversation.com/what-it-means-to-be-black-in-the-american-educational-system-63576.

McCoy, D., C. Luedke, and R. Winkle-Wagner. 2017. Encouraged or weeded out: Perspectives of students of color in the STEM disciplines on faculty interactions. *Journal of College Student Development* 58: 657–673. https://doi.org/10.1353/csd.2017.0052.

McGee, E. O. 2020. *Black, Brown, Bruised: How Racialized STEM Education Stifles Education*. Cambridge, MA: Harvard Education Press.

McGee, E. O., and W. H. Robinson (eds.). 2019. *Diversifying STEM: Multidisciplinary Perspectives on Race and Culture*. New Brunswick, NJ: Rutgers University Press.

3

Early Education as the Pathway to Success: Pre-K to 12

Highlights from the Presentations

- Early debates about Head Start focused on whether it should be more an academic or child/family development program, a debate that continues in different forms today, but building children's agency, self-efficacy, and self-regulation are key (Dr. Gordon).
- The core of learning is internal to a person. When internal images and intentions are on track, the brain will do most of the rest of the work (Dr. Gordon).
- Funding good preschool and supplementation education programs provides a manyfold return on investment (Dr. Malcom).
- Math and science activities in which families learn together reveals the brilliance of the children and strengthens the confidence of parents in their children's success (Mr. Hill).
- Four pillars of mental health are key to academic success, especially for students of color: connection to self, connection to others, sense of purpose, and awareness (Dr. Brizard).
- Access to challenging math and science classes taught by culturally responsive teachers sets students up for future opportunities (Dr. Harris).
- A national survey and focus groups confirm the significant impact of COVID-19 on Black children's education and suggests strategies for transformative change (Dr. Horsford).

Planning committee co-chair Shirley Malcom, Ph.D. (American Association for the Advancement of Science [AAAS]), stressed the importance of "starting early" in helping children along the pathway to a career in science, engineering, or medicine (SEM), referring to the previous Roundtable workshop on K-Graduate education (NASEM, 2022. *Educational Pathways for Black Students in Science, Engineering, and Medicine: Exploring Barriers and Possible Interventions: Proceedings of a Workshop*. Washington, DC: The National Academies Press. https://doi.org/10.17226/26391), as well as Dr. Altha Stewart's keynote (see Chapter 2). That message paves the way to look at solutions systemically, Dr. Malcom suggested, in moderating a session on the topic. The session consisted of a video presentation by Edmund Gordon, Ph.D. (Yale University and Columbia University). Dr. Malcom then engaged in conversation with Kenneth Hill (Chicago Pre-College Science and Engineering Program [ChiS&E]) about innovative programs to reach K–3 students and their parents. A panel followed that consisted of Jean-Claude Brizard, Ph.D. (Digital Promise), Bernard Harris, M.D. (National Math and Science Initiative [NMSI]), and Sonya Douglass Horsford, Ph.D. (Columbia University).

THE IMPORTANCE OF STARTING EARLY

In recognizing the key role of early education on the pathway to success, Dr. Malcom reminded the group that the federal government developed Head Start during the 1960s Great Society period as an early education and care program. She noted it could serve as an example of an existing program to build out to expand pathways for youth. For this reason, she said, she invited Dr. Gordon, one of the creators of Head Start, to discuss the program's early days.

Dr. Gordon recalled that one of the tensions in building Head Start was whether it should be a literacy program or a child/family development program. He favored the latter, but, he recalled, "Some people thought that we people of color were so far behind academically, we should throw money to academics." However, he continued, "Those efforts did not pay off.... As we looked at children in elementary and high school, what we came to realize was that their lack of agency, self-efficacy, and self-regulation were getting in the way."

At this point, he continued, rather than debate the "either/or" of focusing on literacy or development, "let's try to do both, and some more." Providing young children with emotional, social, and relational development is on target, he said, and the research seems to support it. "The core of learning is not external to the person, but internal," he explained. "What you want to do is get internal images and intentions on track, and the human brain will do most of the work if that part is right."

Dr. Malcom pointed out that Head Start continues to operate but not at the level to serve the needs of all who are eligible. She noted that although Dr. Gordon referred to what Head Start could and could not accomplish, research over the years shows the value of early childhood programs. For example, a study of the Perry Preschool Program (Cunha and Heckman, 2009) found a return on investment of between about $7 and $12 for every $1 invested. Additional research shows that money invested in early education pays huge dividends throughout the life course. In looking at systemic models where investments might make a huge difference, she urged "sticking a pin" in the value of early childhood education.

SUPPLEMENTAL EDUCATION

Another area where key investments can make a difference, Dr. Malcom suggested, relates to supplemental education that takes place outside of the classroom. She noted the difficulties in achieving school improvement across the 131,000 public schools in America when control is at state and local levels. Part of the challenge is how to prepare teachers to support education and development of diverse student populations, and how to address students' socioeconomic development needs. Presenters from ChiS&E, Digital Promise, and NMSI placed their programs in the context of strengthening students' science, technology, engineering, and mathematics (STEM) identity. Dr. Malcom noted these programs offer opportunities to scale. Creating system-level change means having things in place that can be replicated, adapted, and offered as possibilities for large numbers of people, she pointed out.

INVOLVING YOUNG CHILDREN AND THEIR FAMILIES

Mr. Hill discussed what he has learned from development of supplemental programs in Detroit and Chicago. He built and ran the Detroit Area Pre-College Engineering Program (DAPCEP)[1] for 28 years and estimates DAPCEP reached 50,000 students over that period. Although most

[1] For more information on DAPCEP, see http://www.dapcep.org.

programs at the time worked with high school students, he explained that DAPCEP targeted middle school students (later going back to Grade 4) so that they could develop the necessary background to take calculus in high school.

When Mr. Hill returned to his hometown of Chicago, he started ChiS&E with K–3 families. "We learned in Detroit that the parents at the lower level really care about their children, love them, and want them to do well," he said. With support from a National Science Foundation grant, ChiS&E provides a hands-on, activity-based science and engineering program for K–3 parents and students.[2] Parents come to realize that their children can understand algebra and scientific concepts in these early years. "The idea is for parents to see that their children are brilliant in ongoing experiences so [that] they believe in their children's ability to excel," he said.

He explained the program aims to (1) create and inspire in both students and parents a quest for math, science, and technology education and experiences beyond K–3; (2) expose parents and students to science and engineering facilities in their communities; (3) provide parents and students opportunities to meet African American, Latino, and other scientists and engineers; (4) involve parents in cyberlearning; (5) provide teacher training for elementary school teachers who will provide the K–3 preengineering curriculum to parents and students; and (6) provide a family support system with information on health, educational opportunities, child psychology, and assistance in working with government agencies.

When asked about outcomes, Mr. Hill reported that 80 percent of the first cohort who started with ChiS&E have selected a STEM career and are going to universities across the country. To Mr. Hill, from a psychological perspective, a key element of success is reinforcing to children and their parents how brilliant they are. "This program is about building parent self-confidence that their children can excel and teaching them to protect [their children] when the system tries to tackle them," he said. Dr. Malcom observed that ChiS&E is counteracting the potential adverse childhood experiences (ACEs) discussed by Dr. Stewart during her keynote (see Chapter 2).

APPLYING THE FOUR PILLARS OF MENTAL HEALTH

Dr. Brizard returned to Dr. Gordon's comments about what the learning sciences show about the importance of self-regulation and executive

---

[2] For more information about this and other ChiS&E efforts, see http://chiprep.org.

function. He stressed that these areas are critical for academic success, and they can be taught, rather than left to accidental discovery. Building on work from the Center for Healthy Minds at the University of Wisconsin–Madison, he referred to four pillars that support mental health, especially for children of color: connection to self, connection to others, sense of purpose, and awareness (Dahl et al., 2020). He continued:

> For someone to engage powerfully in education, identity development is critical, but we know so often, frankly, that the identity of our boys and girls of color is not always developed and sometimes imposed.... The question we have to ask ourselves is, where do we invite students to see themselves? Where do we engage them and honor their perspective?

He noted that while "good stress" helps people navigate and engage in powerful learning, toxic stress impacts the learning centers of the brain, memory, and attention. Many students living in racist systems experience toxic stress and are left to themselves to navigate their coursework and their environments, he stated.

Sense of purpose is critical, he continued. Many programs, including many supplemental programs, do not respect or encourage students' own sense of purpose. Dr. Brizard suggested a great opportunity for supplementary programs is to develop curricula based on the learning sciences and pedagogy, including building on the four pillars. Afterschool programs that can provide resources to children, such as bringing museum resources to the South and West sides of Chicago (an effort in which he is involved), can increase awareness about what exists in the sciences and provide meaningful experiences and potential role models to young people. The Wallace Foundation, he noted, provides support for afterschool programs that are linked to the school-day experience.[3]

Technology can also expand learning, Dr. Brizard concluded. The organization he leads, Digital Promise, sets up 360-degree virtual reality exchanges among other initiatives. As youth in different places talk to each other, their worlds expand.[4] It is now operating globally, including in about 650 schools in 32 states. Teachers and parents are also benefiting, he added.

[3] For more information, see www.wallacefoundation.org.

[4] For more information on Digital Promise, see https://digitalpromise.org/.

EXTENDING ADVANCED MATH AND SCIENCE TO ALL STUDENTS

Dr. Harris said when he speaks with youth, he stands as a physician, astronaut, and entrepreneur, and as an example of what they can do. He agreed with previous speakers about the importance for Black youth to see positive role models instead of negative images in the media.

STEM education is important in ensuring a successful future, he stressed, and "it's also about empowering our students, communities, and parents to believe in them." He urged the "brain trust" present at the workshop to make a difference.

The goal of the National Math and Science Initiative is to advance STEM education to ensure all students, especially those furthest from opportunity, thrive and reach their highest potential as problem solvers and lifelong learners who pursue their passions and tackle the world's toughest challenges, Dr. Harris explained. One way that NMSI does this, he explained, is by identifying and eradicating "STEM deserts" (areas without access to challenging STEM educational opportunities, based on 114 indicators) so that all students have access to the STEM education they need and deserve.[5] NMSI also focuses its work on culturally responsive education and social emotional learning to support teachers and students.

NMSI has reached 2 million students and 65,000 teachers in 1,800 high schools and 45 universities. Its College Readiness Program has led to higher participation and outcomes in Advanced Placement STEM courses (see Figure 3-1). Another program targets military families. A K–12 program offers professional development to working teachers and through teacher preparation programs in 40 universities. STEM majors take courses that prepare them to become classroom teachers. The program is expanding to 11 Historically Black Colleges and Universities (HBCUs) with the goal to increase the number of Black men and women becoming math and science teachers. NMSI is also creating a campaign around the theme "STEM Empowers."

Dr. Harris stresses to students that college is the way to advance. "I wholeheartedly believe that if we can bring education, particularly STEM education, to our communities and to our students, we can make a differ-

---

[5] NMSI had developed an index based on "10 conditions, practices, and outcomes that experts believe are critical to identifying where STEM education is being successfully delivered" and mapped school districts around the country against this index. For more information, see https://www.stemopportunityindex.com.

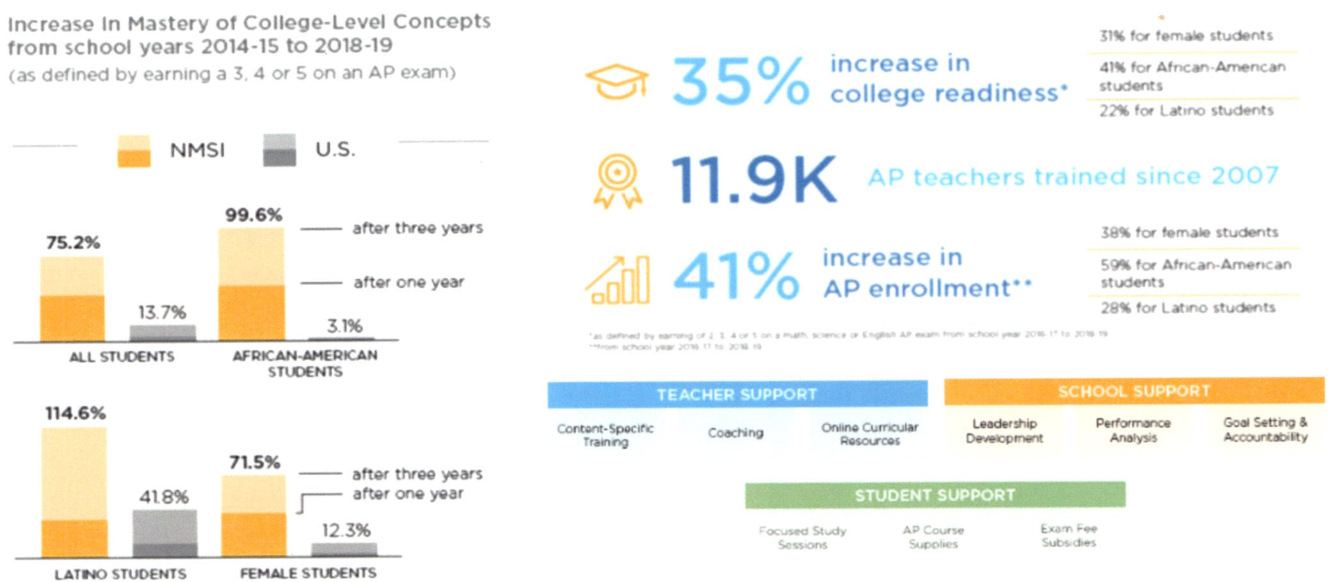

FIGURE 3-1 NMSI College Readiness Programs participation and results.
SOURCE: Bernard Harris, Workshop Presentation, September 14, 2021, based on NMSI data.

ence," he stated. He agreed with the need to help students develop a STEM identity, as well as their own identity. "Our kids need to be reminded how infinite they are," he said. "They need to realize they have the ability to do anything. They have innate abilities and were born for a reason." He said sometimes that gets lost amid economic and social issues. Through positive reinforcement, he concluded, "we enable them in a way like no other."

IMPACT OF COVID-19 ON BLACK STUDENTS

Dr. Horsford summarized a study she led through the Black Education Research Collective in the wake of COVID-19 and systemic racism (Horsford et al., 2021). The intent was to hear directly from students, educators, and caregivers. Two principal research questions were asked: (1) What is the impact of COVID-19 on the education of Black children and youth in the United States? and (2) How should educators and community leaders engage in change and action? It is important to document the challenges but also pivot to what to do about it, she pointed out.

In addition to a national survey, 19 virtual focus groups were held in six metropolitan areas. "The findings were not surprising, but it is stunning to see consistency across communities and stakeholder groups," she commented. These findings included the following:

- COVID-19 and systemic racism have had a disproportionate and traumatic impact on Black students, families, and communities.
- Increased trauma and mental health issues will have major implications for teaching and learning post-COVID-19.
- Schools are ill-equipped to meet the social, emotional, and academic needs of Black students.
- Failed responses to COVID-19, police brutality, and the insurrection at the U.S. Capitol have further reduced trust in schools and public institutions.
- Education leaders and policy makers at the local, state, and federal levels must be held accountable for meeting the educational needs of Black students.

The study's offered solutions include to protect and defend the rights of Black students to receive an appropriate and equitable education in a safe, welcoming, and affirming learning environment; invest in counseling, psychological and mental health services, and support; and provide professional development to teachers and school leaders to meet the needs of Black students. She noted a cultural mismatch in that white women make up 70 to 75 percent of the teacher workforce. She also reflected that the survey and focus group responses show the need to modernize curriculum, pedagogy, and assessment to support affirmative development; to invest in the preparation, cultivation, and mentoring of culturally relevant educators; and to engage Black students, families, educators, researchers, and community leaders as experts and equal partners in advancing educational equity and community transformation for social change. She suggested now is the time for the community to make its needs known and the time for transformative change. While people have been aware of many of these issues, she added, it is important to include it in the evidentiary record.

Dr. Horsford quoted a focus group member who said that "Black education has to be something more along the lines of soul work." This taps into an important theme of the workshop, she observed:

> It is about mind, body, and spirit. For far too long, our education has focused on the academic and cognitive pieces. These are important, but we have to make sure we are focusing on the intellect and how young people strengthen their minds. The mind–body–spirit connections are critical to Black education.

FURTHER REFLECTIONS BY DR. GORDON AND DISCUSSION

Dr. Gordon shared his thoughts as he listened to his fellow panelists. He expressed delight to see the number of people tuned into the problem and capable of doing something about it moving forward, while acknowledging "there are aspects of the problem that are out of our hands, given the history of oppression of people like us." Dr. Gordon recounted that he grew up in rural North Carolina with parents who said he had to try harder because he was Black. "If I just set out to be as good as white folk, I wouldn't make it. I had to be better," he recalled as their lesson to him. The task now, he said, is to corral resources to help and empower young people today. He echoed the idea, as quoted by a member of Dr. Horsford's focus groups, of this being "soul work," and he referred to the power of the "liberating arts and sciences," a concept expressed by scholar W. E. B. Du Bois.

Dr. Gordon said he could summarize his takeaways from the presentations in five expressions: (1) efficacy ("the belief that the task is worth engaging in and I can do it"); (2) agency ("the capacity to look at situations and see what is in my own and my community's best interest"); (3) intellective competence ("knowing, understanding things, and being ready to use knowledge to solve problems"); (4) empowerment ("STEM as a way of empowering students"); and (5) resistance. Related to this latter point, he said, "through all our talks, all of us have found it necessary to call attention to the opposition, and the power of the opposition and the ways in which the opposition is rallying to re-enslave us." The capacity to resist is important, he stressed.

Continuing, he noted that the presenters spoke to paying attention to the mental health of African Americans. He said he distinguished between mental health in the corrective sense, as important as these services are, and mental health in the preventive sense. He elaborated:

> Back in the days when we were trying to create Head Start, we were insisting on building strong families, because it is those things that happen in parent-child relations that lay the first foundations for adequacy, competence, agency, and efficacy, which are the elements of social-emotional development that are so much a part of mental health. Mental health is not just the absence of psychological disturbance, but speaks to the variety of social and emotional competencies that must be increasingly a part of our struggle to move ahead.

As established in Head Start, he said, it is important to start early, not to pour knowledge into kids but to strengthen families to provide the nurturing support and guidance out of which wholesome development comes. Related to supplementary education, he added that efforts that happen outside of school not only are important in themselves but also enable schooling to work. Looking at the relationship between income and education throughout the world, the people who have adequate resources are better educated than those in poverty, he said. "There is something about being well resourced that correlates with good or advanced education. We can't do much about the material resources," he said, but, referring to Dr. Horsford's presentation, "we can go back to the soul work by building the efficacy and agency in young people, which can go a long way to complement Du Bois's notion of learning knowledge for advancement in life."

He concluded that his work is currently directed at a reconceptualization of what it means to have the opportunity to learn. New developments in the learning sciences pay attention to the importance of social and emotional feelings and social relations to learning, he said. For example, a Black child may have trouble performing if she is afraid that in her effort, she will reinforce her teacher's stereotyped belief or bias that she is stupid. That set of feelings may have no reality basis, but it is a force in the mind of that child that limits her capacity. Youngsters must have models and opportunities for success to build a store of confidence and efficacy, he urged. "Out of manifestations of effort we get achievement, and out of the experience of achievement, we gain confidence," Dr. Gordon said.

On the topic of resistance to Black achievements, Mr. Hill commented about the situation in Detroit in which after public school students began excelling at metropolitan-area science fairs, the funding was pulled. Dr. Gordon noted other situations in which success is met with attempts to "pull the rug out." He said the only model to counteract it in a democracy is to resort to democracy itself and have influence in the political arena. This resistance has taken place for eons, Dr. Harris commented. "I have come to the conclusion that we have to be our own affirmative action. Those of us in positions of power, decision making, and leadership must provide support, even economic support because that's what it comes down to. We have to build that wealth within our communities," he stated.

Discussing how to embed racial empowerment into teaching and learning, Dr. Brizard said he agreed with the idea of positioning people of power within communities to protect the investment needed in young people. Cultivating leadership, such as in school systems, universities, and agencies, is critical to supporting the resource flow. For empowerment, he added, "you have to attack it from multiple vantage points. It has to show up in the curriculum and in the pedagogy so there is a hard wiring of the effort," he said. "We have to change the mindset of the people who are in front of our kids through diversity of the teaching and leadership staff and other measures. It is an all-out effort; one lever is not enough."

Related to the mental health ramifications of the "Black tax" for those who excel, Dr. Brizard said he has observed situations in which professionals of color are not just participating in a particular work-related strategy, but having to navigate an environment. Understanding toxic stress is essential, as well as building resilience to navigate systems and pushing the systems to change.

In response to a question, Dr. Horsford said although she could not assume her research is generalizable to rural Black students since it did not take place in those areas, she "has not seen a place yet where Black students are being educated to the best of their ability." That signals the need for systemic change, she added. "We have focused on assimilating to the system and tinkering around the edges, but I do think we have an opportunity to really rebuild it," she said.

Dr. Malcom concluded that K–12 education is "where we will lose the most people if we don't do something about it, but also where we have the least amount of control" because of how the formal education system is structured. She noted the presenters' solutions stressed the importance of early and supplemental education, building community, and reengaging around issues.

REFERENCES

Dahl, C., C. Wilson-Mendenhall, and R. Davidson. 2020. The plasticity of well-being: A training-based framework for the cultivation of human flourishing. *Proceedings of the National Academy of Sciences* 117(51): 32197–32206. https://doi.org/10.1073/pnas.2014859117.

Cunha, F., and J. J. Heckman. 2009. The Economics and Psychology of Inequality and Human Development. *Journal of the European Economic Association* 7(2):320–364. https://doi.org/10.1162/jeea.2009.7.2-3.320.

Horsford, S. D., L. Cabral, C. Touloukian, S. Parks, P. A. Smith, C. McGhee, F. Qadir, D. Lester, and J. Jacobs. 2021. *Black Education in the Wake of COVID-19 and Systemic Racism: Where Do We Go from Here?* https://www.tc.columbia.edu/media/centers/berc/Final-BERC-COVID-Report-20July2021.pdf.

4

Higher Education and Institutional Changes

Highlights from the Presentations

- Keys to success to increase Black representation in medical and other health professional training include frequent and meaningful advisement sessions with students; training and support of college pre-health advisors, K–12 teachers, and college faculty; summer research and clinical shadowing opportunities; mentorship programs, career and academic support and guidance, and enrichment workshops; standardized test preparation through pipeline programs; personal and professional development opportunities; clinical and research exposure with renowned experts; and tuition scholarships and scholarships for travel to scientific and medical conferences (Dr. Montgomery Rice).
- The Fisk-Vanderbilt Master's-to-Ph.D. Bridge Program begins with a holistic admission process to enter the program; once students are at Vanderbilt, they capitalize on the culture and traditions of Fisk to build community (Dr. Stassun).
- Rather than rely on "one perfect mentor," a network of mentors who can meet different needs may be more beneficial (Dr. Stassun).
- The Meyerhoff Scholars Program, begun at the University of Maryland, Baltimore County in 1987, is 7 times more likely

to produce students who pursue graduate STEM degrees than high-achieving students who do not participate in such a program (Dr. Summers).

- The model, with its emphasis on high expectations and team building, has been successfully adapted in at least three other universities (Dr. Summers).
- To unleash Black women's "STEM Superpowers," Spelman College identifies high-impact practices to build cohorts and learning communities, cultural relevance and social responsiveness to provide agency, and critical race theory and Black feminist thought to foster STEM identity (Dr. Jackson).
- Building cohorts of Black female undergraduates with the intentionality to pursue Ph.D. degrees creates bonds that last up the career ladder (Dr. Jackson).

Planning committee co-chair Evelynn Hammonds, Ph.D. (Harvard University), moderated a session to discuss changes at colleges and universities to improve access, success, and well-being. Panelists included Valerie Montgomery Rice, M.D. (Morehouse School of Medicine [MSM]); Keivan Stassun, Ph.D. (Vanderbilt and Fisk Universities); Mike Summers, Ph.D. (University of Maryland, Baltimore County [UMBC]); and Kimberly Jackson, Ph.D. (Spelman College). In addition to helping Black female and male students, Dr. Hammonds said, they have worked to change the institutional landscape of the schools and communities.

MOREHOUSE SCHOOL OF MEDICINE: INNOVATING AGAINST THE ODDS

Dr. Montgomery Rice began by calling attention to the title of her presentation, noting, "We are *still* innovating against the odds." She recently published a commentary in *JAMA* in which she pointed out that despite the creation of 14 new medical schools over the past decade, the number of underrepresented minorities (URMs) in medicine has not significantly increased (Montgomery Rice, 2021). Every school includes diversity in their mission statements, she observed, but they have not lived up to their missions. She pointed out the greatest number of URMs in medicine, including African Americans, continues to come from Historically Black Colleges and Universities (HBCUs) and minority-serving institutions. Black men make up less than 3 percent of positions in medical school, she added, "and this requires immediate action."

Dr. Montgomery Rice highlighted several efforts at Morehouse School of Medicine to strengthen the applicant pool. It is important to conceptualize the work as "more of a pathway than a pipeline, and that pathway begins at K [kindergarten] through 5," she said. Echoing previous presenters, she stressed elementary school is when individuals begin to set their future course. Scientific enrichment programs in the early years make a difference, she underscored, and commented, "This is one of the low-hanging fruits that we can do."

MSM is partnering with the American Association of Medical Colleges and others to develop a national repository where people can learn the objectives, metrics, and toolkits of existing programs, rather than "reinvent the wheel."[1] As an example, MSM's S.T.E.A.M. Academy has programs for grades 4 to 8 and for 9 to 12.[2] "It's about improving their problem solving, critical thinking, and creativity," she explained, noting that the arts are included. One lesson of the pandemic has been to show that virtual learning can be hands-on, and hybrid programs will continue to reach more students, she added.

The First Look community services project introduces high school and undergraduate students to what is involved in pursuing scientific and health careers, she explained. In addition, the Undergraduate Health Sciences Academy is a very intentional program to increase the number of undergraduates from the Atlanta University Center Consortium to enter careers in the health professions and biomedical sciences. Thirty students, 10 from each school (Morehouse, Clark Atlanta, and Spelman), have summer research programs, mentors, and other support. Outcomes include 88 percent retention in staying in science fields, and 82 percent going on to medical, physician assistants, dental, or doctoral programs. A master of science in medical sciences serves as MSM's postbaccalaureate program. She called attention to its success rate in which from 80 to 100 percent are accepted into professional or doctoral programs after participating in this "graduate academic enhancer."

"We understand that it can't just be on the four HBCUs to graduate Black and Brown students. We are not trying to absorb by any means the

---

[1] For more information, see https://www.msm.edu/Community/commonspirithealth/index.php

[2] For more information, see https://www.msm.edu/Education/PipelinePrograms/STEAMacademy.php.

other 152 medical schools. But we can do more," Dr. Montgomery Rice said.[3] In 2020, MSM and Common Spirit Health, one of the nation's largest nonprofit health-care systems, announced a partnership to train more Black physicians.[4] Over the next 5 to 7 years, she reported, MSM will establish new regional medical campuses and graduate education sites to involve 300 additional students per year in residency programs, with the intentionality to target Black and Brown students. In addition, an investment from the Bloomberg Philanthropies to the four HBCU medical schools is being used to defray student debt that impacts many Black and Brown students and physicians.

Dr. Montgomery Rice closed with what she sees as the keys to success to increase the number of Black health professionals:

- Frequent and meaningful advisement sessions with students
- Training and support to college pre-health advisors, K–12 teachers, and college faculty to help them understand the needs and contexts of students
- Summer research and clinical shadowing opportunities for students
- Mentorship programs, career and academic support and guidance, and enrichment workshops
- Standardized test preparation through pipeline programs
- Personal and professional development opportunities
- Clinical and research exposure with renowned experts in their disciplines
- Tuition scholarships and scholarships for travel to scientific and medical conferences

FISK-VANDERBILT MASTER'S-TO-PH.D. BRIDGE PROGRAM: FROM ADMISSIONS TO COMMUNITY

Dr. Stassun shared lessons from building and running the Fisk-Vanderbilt Master's-to-Ph.D. Bridge Program. He explained that he helped create the program in his first year as a Vanderbilt assistant professor in 2004

---

[3] In addition to MSM, these medical schools include Charles R. Drew University of Medicine and Science, Howard University College of Medicine, and Meharry Medical College.

[4] For more information, see https://www.msm.edu/Community/commonspirithealth/index.php.

and, to date, about 150 students, 90 percent of whom are URMs, have participated. Fisk University is now the nation's largest producer of master's degrees by African American students in physics and materials science, and Vanderbilt has become one of the largest producers of Ph.D.'s by URMs across the physical sciences.

In setting up the program to increase representation, a major barrier identified was over-reliance on standardized test scores in graduate admissions. Traditionally, Ph.D.-granting institutions manage their graduate science, technology, engineering, and mathematics (STEM) admissions through a form of triage, with Graduate Record Examination (GRE) scores having an outsized influence on which applicants are considered in the next stage. Stassun and a colleague published an article in *Nature* (Miller and Stassun, 2014) that showed the powerful negative correlation between race, ethnicity, and GRE scores. The Fisk-Vanderbilt program instead shifted to a holistic review process. Multiple factors create a fair and consistent review, without an overreliance on test scores, to include undergraduate courses, perseverance, setting and pursuing long-term goals, preparedness, and potential.

Once the admissions barrier is overcome and students enter the program, a sense of community must be built, Dr. Stassun continued. Vanderbilt's partnership with Fisk had to consist of more than good intentions to provide real community, he said. As students transition to the Ph.D. programs at Vanderbilt, they still capitalize on the community and tradition of Fisk. The program has also rethought mentorship to provide multiple sources for students to meet their different needs. For example, he noted he cannot be a student's only mentor, especially for a student who needs access to top labs and networks that he as an astrophysicist cannot provide. He noted the science of effective mentorship in STEM indicates the value of going beyond a dyad and the myth of "one perfect mentor" to move toward mentoring networks in which mentees have access to multiple mentors to be successful (NASEM, 2019).

UNIVERSITY OF MARYLAND, BALTIMORE COUNTY: MEYERHOFF MODEL

Dr. Summers has been on the UMBC faculty since 1987, the same year that Freeman A. Hrabowski III, Ph.D., joined the faculty. While experimenting for success is always needed, Dr. Summers said, the experience at UMBC pioneered by Dr. Hrabowski has worked extremely well. Dr.

Summers described the Meyerhoff Scholars model at UMBC and highlighted its successful adaptation at other universities.

At UMBC, the Meyerhoff Scholars model involves like-minded high achievers, 70 percent of whom are URMs, Dr. Summers explained, and they experience intrusive support, high expectations, and cohort learning. A summer bridge program is essential, and students learn how to support each other by working in teams. High exposure on the predominantly white campus is also required, he added. For example, in a large chemistry lecture hall, Meyerhoff Scholars are expected to arrive 15 minutes early, sit together at the front, and engage with the professor. This raises the expectations of faculty about Meyerhoff students and promotes climate change.

Of the 1,490 Meyerhoff participants to date, 71 percent have been URMs, with 91 percent retained in STEM. Among the 930 who have pursued graduate or professional degrees, 312 Ph.D.'s have been awarded (82 percent URMs), 59 M.D.'s/Ph.D.'s have been awarded (90 percent URMs), and 265 STEM master's degrees have been awarded (86 percent URMs). In addition, 258 (81 percent URMs) are currently enrolled in graduate schools. Most of the underrepresented students are African American, he said.

Research counters the assumption that because the program recruits high-achievers, the students would have done just as well without the program. Researchers compared outcomes between Meyerhoff Scholars and students who were accepted into the program but chose to attend another institution. Dr. Summers reported that students who went elsewhere graduate with similar GPAs (grade point averages), but they are half as likely to graduate with STEM degrees and 7 times less likely to complete STEM graduate degrees than Meyerhoff Scholars (Maton et al., 2009, 2012). A broader impact on society includes such leaders as Kizzmekia Corbett, Ph.D., a leader in COVID-19 vaccine development; former Surgeon General Jerome Adams; and National Institutes of Health (NIH) award recipient Kafui Dzirasa, Ph.D. (a speaker later in the workshop; see Chapter 6). More than 40 tenured or tenure-track faculty are UMBC Meyerhoff graduates, he added.

Dr. Summers noted the outcomes have been replicated elsewhere. The Howard Hughes Medical Institute (HHMI) supported partnerships with the University of North Carolina (UNC) and Pennsylvania State University (Penn State), which he noted have different characteristics than UMBC. Outcomes almost immediately met or exceeded Meyerhoff outcomes in terms of STEM retention, 4-year graduation rates, Ph.D. matriculation, and minority participation (Sto Domingo et al., 2019). He noted that

HHMI and other grants, as well as institutional commitments, are necessary to fund the program. Institutional funds do not necessarily mean new money, but rather a refocusing of existing scholarship funds to support the program. Both the UNC and Penn State programs have begun to build dedicated endowment as well.

Dr. Summers has also been involved in a program started in 2012 by the chemistry faculty at his alma mater, University of West Florida. Beginning with informal meetings with students to talk about diversity, the program is now supported by NIH and the National Science Foundation (NSF), and the institution recently provided $500,000 from its institutional budget to move the program across the campus. Although it does not have all the elements of the Meyerhoff Scholars Program, it has had 70 percent URM STEM retention. Sixty-three percent of the students are pursuing Ph.D. or M.D./Ph.D. degrees, the majority in the nation's top 25 graduate programs.

In conclusion, Dr. Summers said, large numbers of minority students are interested in STEM, but few are retained. High achievers will succeed without this support, but are less likely to pursue a STEM Ph.D. Institutional partnerships work well. Strong alliances with like-minded colleagues can be built with positive messaging and data.

SPELMAN COLLEGE: PROMOTING SUCCESS AND WELL-BEING AT A WOMEN'S COLLEGE

Dr. Jackson spoke about work to diversify the STEM pathway and advance equity in STEM for Black women. In addition to being ranked the nation's top HBCU by *U.S. News & World Report*, she called attention to Spelman's top ranking across all institutions in other measures related to teaching and innovation. She said Spelman is ranked first in producing African American women who go on to earn Ph.D.'s in science-related fields and first overall in where Black science and engineering doctorate recipients earned their bachelor's degrees, according to NSF data.

Several years ago, Dr. Jackson reported, faculty from across the campus came together to discuss the "intellectual table" that is set for students. Essential elements they identified included high-impact practices to build cohorts and learning communities; cultural relevance and social responsiveness to provide agency; and critical race theory and Black feminist thought to foster STEM identity. Around 2013, she and fellow professor Leyte Winfield, Ph.D., created the Women of Color Legacy Project. They won an NIH planning grant to develop the tenets of the project with the objective of being transformative, systemic, catalytic, synergistic, and unique. The project recognizes a multipronged cycle beginning with early investment in middle school and high school students through alumnae and professionals, Dr. Jackson explained.

Although the project did not receive full NIH funding, the planning grant allowed for discussions about how to cultivate "superwomen" in recognition that Spelman is uniquely poised to transform the current STEM landscape. She and Dr. Winfield published on the types of practices used by Spelman faculty, including authentic research experiences, effective mentoring, and innovative and impactful curricula (Jackson and Winfield, 2014). An important part of mentoring is to help young women embrace their identity, she added.

Dr. Jackson stressed that the work is centered on an empowerment, rather than a deficit, model. She explained:

> Our goal is not to fix our students at all. We embrace their identity and cultivate their success. We recognize they are unique, we acknowledge their potential, we support sisterhood, we highlight Black female scholars, and we create opportunities because we believe that if you can see yourself, you can become whatever you want to be.

Spelman also separated out parts of the Women of Color Legacy proposal for implementation. Dr. Jackson and biology colleague Menteweb Ayalew, Ph.D., developed a program called Living and Learning in an Interdisciplinary Networked Community of STEM (LINCS) Scholars. Begun 6 years ago with no funding, it developed from learning that many students leave STEM fields because of isolation and lack of support. Through LINCS, cohorts with strong and lasting bonds move together up the academic and career ladder and leverage peer–peer and peer–outside networks. The community is now part of Spelman's Social Justice Fellows Program in recognition that occupying a unique space at the multiple intersections of race, gender, and STEM is a social justice issue. The program creates synergies with other programs on campus and now has its fourth cohort of 21 sophomores and juniors with a declared interest in pursuing a Ph.D. degree. Dr. Jackson said the next step is to engage in hard conversations at the departmental level related to vision, metrics, and teaching strategies. In 2021–2022, the focus is to leverage what they have learned to tackle racialized issues in STEM.

DISCUSSION

Dr. Hammonds asked the presenters about how to ensure sustainability and funding of programs. Dr. Montgomery Rice suggested approaching NIH and other federal agencies. She also urged more leeway so that HBCUs with a track record can use the funding they receive for sustainability. If these programs were endowed, the pathway could continue and additional fundraising could take place. In addition to public support, Dr. Summers added many large majority schools focus on raising money for athletics, and there is a large pool of money that could be reinvested in other areas. It is important to have leadership who sees these programs as a priority in using institutional resources.

Dr. Stassun emphasized a role for partnerships, especially when academic strategic planning identifies diversity as an important goal. He also noted that federal agencies such as NSF like the idea of partnerships to provide glue between institutions to enable students' successful transitions. However, partnerships must be equitable, Dr. Jackson stressed. Spelman is often approached to be a partner but without equitable funding or power sharing. Dr. Stassun agreed and noted federal agencies can exert leverage, such as requiring the principal investigator be at the minority institution or that articulated outcomes include capacity building for an MSI (math and science initiative) partner. "The dollars have to flow in ways that benefit the students, the faculty, and the institutions," he said.

In concluding the session, Dr. Hammonds commented, "It's really important to understand that there have been institutions that have successfully been addressing the kinds of psychological, behavioral, individual but also group-level interventions that help our students succeed. We can build on the programs we heard about." Dr. Pinn added that these achievements show evidence of action. "We often put things into committees and discuss or do more research, but it's time now for action to happen. Each of the institutions have put in place something and are moving forward, and we need to learn from those examples," she said.

REFERENCES

Jackson, K. M., and L. L. Winfield. 2014. Realigning the crooked room: Spelman claims a space for African American women in STEM. *Peer Review: Emerging Trends and Key Debates in Undergraduate Education* 16(2): 9–12. https://www.ncbi.nlm.nih.gov/pmc/articles/PMC4280840.

Maton, K. I., M. R. Sto Domingo, K. E. Stolle-McAllister, J. L. Zimmerman, and F. A. Hrabowski, III. 2009. Enhancing the number of African-Americans who pursue STEM PhDs: Meyerhoff Scholarship Program outcomes, processes, and individual behaviors. *Journal of Women and Minorities in Science and Engineering* 15(1): 15–37.

Maton, K. I., S. A. Pollard, T. V. McDougall Weise, and F. A. Hrabowski. 2012. The Meyerhoff Scholars Program: A strengths-based, institution-wide approach to increasing diversity in science, technology, engineering, and mathematics. *Mount Sinai Journal of Medicine* 79(5): 610–623.

Miller, C., and K. Stassun. 2014. A test that fails. *Nature* 510: 303–304.

Montgomery Rice, V. 2021. Diversity in Medical Schools: A Much-Needed New Beginning. *Journal of the American Medical Association* 325(1):23–24. https://doi.org/10.1001/jama.2020.21576.

NASEM (National Academies of Sciences, Engineering, and Medicine). 2019. *The Science of Effective Mentorship in STEMM.* Washington, DC: The National Academies Press. https://doi.org/10.17226/25568.

Sto Domingo, M. R., S. Sharp, A. Freeman, T. Freeman Jr., K. Harmon, M. Wiggs, V. Sathy, A. T. Panter, L. Oseguera, S. Sun, M. E. Williams, J. Templeton, C. L. Folt, E. J. Barron, F. A. Hrabowski III, K. I. Maton, M. Crimmins, C. R. Fisher, and M. F. Summers. 2019. Replicating Meyerhoff of inclusive excellence in STEM. *Science* 364 (6438): 335–337.

5

Bringing Systemic Changes through Important Sectors of Influence

Highlights from the Presentations

- The Commonwealth Fund bases its systems-level health equity goal on three focus areas: advancing health equity at the systems level requires dismantling racism in care delivery; using policy to bring about equitable access; and changing culture, belief, and attitudes (Dr. Zephyrin).
- Comprehensive primary health care, to include mental health care, can be achieved through multidisciplinary provider teams, integration of digital health tools, community engagement, and integration of health and social needs (Dr. Zephyrin).
- The NIH UNITE Initiative was launched to address structural racism within NIH and the extramural community (Dr. Bernard).
- UNITE has five interacting work streams: (1) understand stakeholder experiences; (2) fund new research; (3) improve the NIH culture and structure for equity, inclusion, and excellence; (4) promote transparency, communication, and accountability; and (5) create extramural research ecosystem changes (Dr. Bernard).
- Rigorous research is needed to understand the collective impact of institutional forces on psychological distress (Dr. Marrett).

- There is an imperative for collaborations across agencies if the nation is to profit from models that center on systems and not just individuals (Dr. Marrett).
- Health plans can be leaders in advancing health equity by focusing on data analytics, creating a skilled workforce, being nimble about innovation, and addressing implicit bias (Dr. Olayiwola).
- Taking a hard and humble look at the data is important in understanding challenges and developing effective solutions (Dr. Olayiwola).

Garth Graham, M.D., M.P.H. (Google, Inc.), moderated a panel on bringing systemic changes to influencers in the private and public sectors. He stressed the need to identify the "10,000-foot mental health issues" that can undermine career advancement for Black and Brown men and women in science, technology, engineering, and mathematics (STEM). The panel consisted of Laurie Zephyrin, M.D., M.P.H., MBA (Commonwealth Fund); Marie Bernard, M.D. (National Institutes of Health [NIH]); Cora Marrett, Ph.D. (University of Wisconsin–Madison); and Nwando Olayiwola, M.D., M.P.H. (Humana).

ADVANCING HEALTH EQUITY AT THE POLICY LEVEL

Dr. Zephyrin began with a macro-level picture of how health policy can lead to systems change. A high-performing health-care system cannot be created without advancing health equity, she stressed. The goal of the Commonwealth Fund is to eliminate unequal treatment, experience, and outcomes in health and health care for people of color by dismantling systemic racism in health-care policy and practice. Three focus areas underpin the framework to achieve this goal: dismantling racism in care delivery; using policy to bring about equitable access; and changing culture, beliefs, and attitudes.[1]

Dr. Zephyrin underscored that strategies for health-care delivery system change involve what happens not only within the walls of a health-care institution, but also in the broader community. Strategies include diversifying and training the workforce; engaging with partners; and dis-

[1] For more information on the Commonwealth Fund, see https://www.commonwealthfund.org.

aggregating data to measure outcomes, experience, and quality over time. The Commonwealth Fund is committed to creating an ecosystem and roadmap as organizations develop their antiracism agendas, she explained. Strategies for health policy change extend to all sectors of society:

> Policy helps drive systems change and individual actions on the ground. Federal and state policy makers can adopt policies and procedures that can advance racial equity and address racism in health care. This can include incorporating equity in value-based care arrangements to incentivize payment to ensure that health systems are advancing health equity and that policies are achieving intended outcomes.

Related to the workshop focus, Dr. Zephyrin pointed out that comprehensive primary health care can make mental health care available and accessible. Health-care fragmentation is reduced through multidisciplinary provider teams; integration of digital health tools; community engagement; and integration between physical health, behavioral health, and health-related social needs.

Policy makers and health systems leaders have important roles to implement change, she concluded. They can help use program and policy levers; promote systemic change and antiracism in health policy and payment models; center community-based solutions; promote institutional change through new models of care in delivery systems; measure the progress of health-care delivery systems toward achieving equity; and disseminate resources on how systemic racism manifests in health-care systems.

ADDRESSING RACISM AT NIH AND IN THE EXTRAMURAL COMMUNITY

The NIH UNITE Initiative came about in 2020 in recognition of the ongoing reality of racial injustice and responsibility of everyone to address it, reported Dr. Bernard. Discussion among NIH Institute and Center (IC) directors identified initial issues to undertake. Self-assembled affinity groups, including a group of early-career scientists, came forward to "speak truth to power," she said. They brought data and case studies to the attention of NIH Director Francis Collins, M.D., Ph.D., and Principal Deputy Director Lawrence Tabak, D.D.S., Ph.D., that showed that the racism seen in society existed at NIH. Senior scientists of color and an already-established Anti-Harassment Steering Committee reinforced the message that led to the next steps. "We have arrived at a shared commitment to address structural racism," said Dr. Bernard. "We must not allow this pivotal moment to pass."

Initial issues identified include ensuring that biomedical research, and the administrative system that supports it, is devoid of hostility grounded in race, sex, or other federally protected characteristics, Dr. Bernard said. This means a commitment to delineate elements both within NIH and in the extramural community that lead to a lack of personnel inclusiveness, equity, and diversity. All ideas must be given an equal and fair review, without regard to current dogma, precedents, or who presents the idea. As COVID-19 made clear, health disparities and inequities persist, and it is essential to redress their fundamental causes and identify research programs and effective interventions.

Formally announced on February 26, 2021, the NIH UNITE Initiative consists of five interacting work streams: (1) understanding stakeholder experiences through listening and sharing; (2) new research on health disparities, minority health, and health equity; (3) improving the NIH culture and structure for equity, inclusion, and excellence; (4) transparency, communication, and accountability with internal and external stakeholders; and (5) extramural research ecosystem changes in policy, culture, and structure to promote workforce diversity.

The groups responsible for each area regularly report on recommendations and progress, with the first such report in June 2021. She noted the NIH director published an apology to "those individuals in the biomedical research enterprise who have endured disadvantages due to structural racism."[2] NIH also committed to aggressively implementing approaches to address the "Ginther Gap," and enhance portfolio diversity. She explained that the term stems from research published by Donna Ginther, Ph.D., and colleagues that documented that Black and African American scientists receive disproportionately fewer R01 grants than white applicants (Ginther et al., 2011). The research led to the establishment of the position that Dr. Bernard currently holds, the chief officer for scientific workforce diversity. Data since then have shown progress, but a gap in success rates and overall numbers of Black and Hispanic applicants still exists. "This is what we are committed to work on until you cannot predict based upon a person's

[2] For the full statement and other information, see https://www.nih.gov/ending-structural-racism.

demographics the likelihood that a researcher will be successful with NIH funding," she said.

NIH launched a multi-phased, tiered, and integrated Common Fund Initiative to support transformative health disparities research initiatives. Two Common Funding Opportunity Announcements (FOAs) were released in March 2021 that initially commit up to $24 million to this research.[3] A robust NIH-wide commitment to support an FOA by the National Institute on Minority Health and Health Disparities on the health impacts of structural racism was also announced, with commitments of up to $30.8 million from other ICs.

Going forward, priorities include additional funding for research on health disparities, minority health, and health equity research for the four ICs that have the most underrepresented minority researchers applying for R01 funding; FOAs in other ICs; programs to spur changes in institutional culture change (including Faculty Institutional Recruitment for Sustainable Transformation, or FIRST);[4] and support for the Science Education Partnership Award (targeted at K–12 students) and minority-serving institutions, including Historically Black Colleges and Universities.

Dr. Bernard called attention to posting of a notice about how to report harassment or discrimination to NIH, published in August 2021. She concluded that the strength of the program is its systemic and comprehensive effort (Collins et al., 2021).

RESEARCH IMPERATIVES FOR SYSTEMS CHANGE

The mission of the National Science Foundation (NSF) is to keep the nation at the cutting edge of innovation and to attend to the education of the populace. Dr. Marrett drew on her experience in NSF leadership positions to summarize NSF's efforts to fulfill that mission and discuss ways in which the workshop can help NSF further strengthen its contributions through an equity lens.

Given the focus of the workshop on broader contexts for psychological well-being, Dr. Marrett expressed dismay that only limited research has been conducted on the impact of institutional forces on psychological dis-

---

[3] As of this writing, the deadline for FY 2021 submission has passed and applications are under review.

[4] This program provides an estimated $241 million over 9 years. For more information, see NIH Faculty Institutional Recruitment for Sustainable Transformation (FIRST) program at https://www.commonfund.nih.gov/first.

tress. "We know a lot more about the consequences of particular kinds of relationships or dislocations than the larger socio-cultural context and systemic forces," she observed. Examples of this more specific research include the consequences of violence or of COVID-19 on psychological distress. She noted that support across several NSF directorates recognizes that the well-being of a population can be indicated by more than what one sees at the level of the individual. For example, the Engineering Directorate is funding a study on the effect of mental wellness on retention in engineering programs. As another example, the ADVANCE Program, which focuses on promoting women in STEM fields, has been on the NSF agenda for some time.[5] When it was launched in 2001, there was discussion about whether to focus on individuals or institutions. While the initial decision was to try to do both, the institutional emphasis came to prevail over time.

Dr. Marrett called for ways to bring together entities that are potentially related to each other to expand the agenda to change systems. She elaborated:

> The research that is available tends to be less expansive and provides far less coverage of the Black population than might be warranted. We need to attend to the question of greater collaboration. NSF is influential but cannot be the sole source for unraveling complexities. Other national agencies, especially within the sphere of health care, play critical roles. That means there is an imperative for collaborations if the nation is to profit from models that center on systems and not just individuals.

She also suggested that health plans and other organizations share resources and ideas to produce outcomes for conducting research, delivering services, finding solutions, and mobilizing amid complexity. Influencers, including NSF, can contribute to the building of capacity, advancement of scholarship, and provision of resources to shape policies. She urged rigorous research on some issues emerging out of the workshop, such as the value of cultural wealth.

---

[5] For more information on the ADVANCE Program, see https://www.nsf.gov/crssprgm/advance/.

OPPORTUNITIES FOR HEALTH PLANS

Dr. Olayiwola began by expressing appreciation to Dr. Marrett for highlighting that health plans have a role to advance health equity. When she began her position at Humana, she said, she published an article on what health plans can do to use their domains of influence in tackling structural racism and moving to a more equitable health-care ecosystem (Olayiwola, 2021). She said health plans can be leaders to address the social and structural determinants of health; deliver comprehensive clinical care, especially for those who have been marginalized; provide an enhanced consumer journey; build capacity through academic partnerships and workforce development; and leverage capital to empower community engagement and partnerships. It requires a focus on data analytics and creating a skilled workforce, being nimble about innovation, and implicit bias (see Figure 5-1).

Black and Hispanic workers remain highly underrepresented in the STEM workforce, she reminded the group, with challenges both in entering and advancing in the field. Intersectionality compounds disparities, she continued, quoting poet and activist Audre Lord, who stated, "There is no thing as a single-issue struggle because we do not live single-issue lives." For example, scientists and engineers with disabilities have higher unemployment, receive fewer grants and other support, and were only 1 percent of medical students in 2019. This inequity is more pronounced for individuals of color who also have disabilities. Dr. Olayiwola reflected on the role of health plans like Humana:

> Our industry in the payer space has a great imperative to not only develop the pipeline of Black men and Black women that enter into the STEM professions but also stay in the pipeline. The areas where we should focus on, and we have the opportunity to focus on, are in the early spaces … educational opportunities, mentoring and career advancement, and removing barriers and addressing biases in our practices.

She described several Humana-supported programs for pregnant women, young girls, and other populations. Along with organizations, Humana supports the OneTen Coalition to upskill, hire, and promote 1 million Black Americans over 10 years. Other investments address food and housing insecurity to remove barriers to mobility and education. The organization is also working on policies and practices within its own workforce.

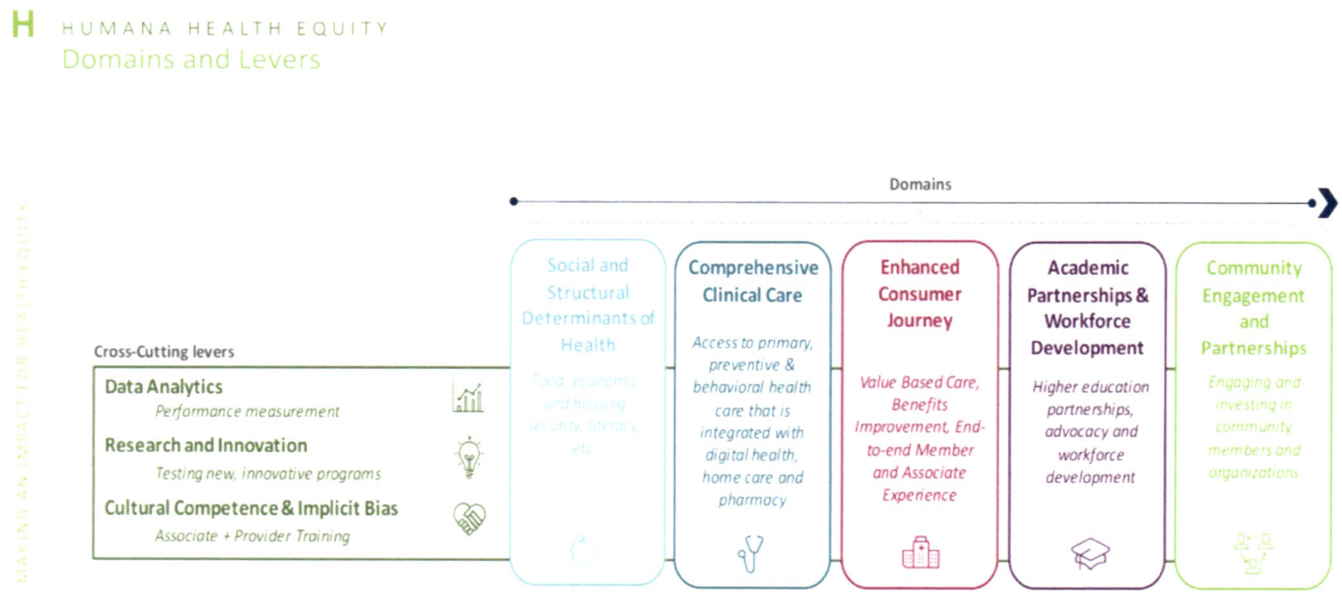

FIGURE 5-1 Opportunities for health plans in advancing health equity.
SOURCE: Nwando Olayiwola, Workshop Presentation, September 14, 2021.

"It's time for health organizations to lean into our role and our opportunity," Dr. Olayiwola concluded. "If health plans can align on this kind of work and imperative, we have a lot of data, influence, and members. We can make a difference."

DISCUSSION

Dr. Graham commented that structural racism has been hundreds of years in the making, and posed the question about the levers to pull given this complexity. Dr. Bernard suggested that embedding changes in the federal government may have a ripple effect. Dr. Marrett pointed out that the National Academies of Sciences, Engineering, and Medicine has placed the issue high on its agenda, and she urged taking advantage of the National Academies' stature in scientific and policy-making circles. Dr. Zephyrin also pointed to the importance of policy making because "policies drive incentives and help drive action." Dr. Olayiwola agreed, but she also urged taking a "hard and humble look at the data" to understand progress and gaps. She commented that while health plans compete on a number of fronts, addressing the social determinants of health is an area for strengthening and collaboration.

In terms of federal support, Dr. Marrett and Dr. Bernard both urged not waiting to respond to funding announcements or requests for proposals but to be proactive in contacting NSF, NIH, and other agencies.

REFERENCES

Collins, F. S., A. B. Adams, C. Aklin, T. K. Archer, M. A. Bernard, E. Boone, J. Burklow, M. K. Evans, S. Jackson, A. C. Johnson, J. Lorsch, M. R. Lowden, A. M. Nápoles, A. E. Ordóñez, R. Rivers, V. Rucker, T. Schwetz, J. A. Segre, L. A. Tabak, M. Webb Hooper, C. Wolinetz, and NIH UNITE. 2021. Affirming NIH's commitment to addressing structural racism in the biomedical research enterprise. *Cell* 184(12): 3075–3079. https://doi.org/10.1016/j.cell.2021.05.014.

Ginther, D. K., W. T. Schaffer, J. Schnell, B. Masimore, F. Liu, L. L. Haakand, and R. Kington. 2011. Race, ethnicity, and NIH research awards. *Science* 333(6045): 1015–1019. https://doi.org/10.1126/science.1196783.

Olayiwola, J. N. 2021. Five keys to realizing health equity in U.S. health plans. *Health Affairs Forefront* (blog). https://doi.org/10.1377/hblog20210518.626084.

6

Development and Implementation of Equity-Based Strategies

Highlights from the Presentations

- In addition to the social determinants of health, the political determinants of health can effect change (Ms. Davis).
- Who makes the policies is also important. It is important for funders to look at how decisions are made and if they are being made equitably (Ms. Davis).
- Because philanthropy is not beholden to investors, shareholders, or other political forces, it can leverage capital in innovative ways (Mr. Gill).
- How to build a more inclusive and equitable scientific enterprise is a phenomenal place for independent capital to be used (Mr. Gill).
- Intellect is distributed evenly across the population. But unless the human tendency to prefer "sameness" is challenged, the talent that resides in much of the population will remain untapped (Dr. Dzirasa).
- A principal investigator experiment with long-term funding is needed to figure out what has worked nationally and how to scale what has worked (Dr. Dzirasa).

Continuing the conversation about the role of policy in creating system change, Sudip Parikh, Ph.D. (American Association for the Advancement of Science [AAAS]), moderated a panel that looked at the nexus of science, policy, and business. He posed a series of questions to Kafui Dzirasa, M.D., Ph.D. (Duke University); Michellene Davis, Esq. (National Medical Fellowships, Inc.); and Samsher Singh Gill (Doris Duke Charitable Foundation).

OVERCOMING PERSISTENT BARRIERS

Before becoming president and CEO of National Medical Fellowships (NMF), Ms. Davis worked in a leadership position at a large academic health center in New Jersey. She reflected on that experience in discussing barriers to equity and a more diverse health workforce:

> We can call it strategic tension, we can call it the interest in keeping the status quo, we can call it what we like, but we know not just that structural or systemic racism exists within institutions, but that, quite frankly, white supremacist culture in organizations helps to keep it as embedded as it has always been.

In her view, until opportunities for diverse physician-leaders improve, that "strategic tension" will remain in place. In her new position at NMF, she said she hears about the experiences of students who have been discouraged from pursuing medicine, see few role models, experience lack of economic and social capital, and have little access to opportunities. Ms. Davis added her background in politics serves her well in advancing health equity because it has made her aware not just of social determinants of health but also of political determinants of health created by laws, regulations, and policy.

Dr. Dzirasa stressed the importance of centering on both overt and systemic racism. In engineering terms, he elaborated, overt racism stems from a policy in which two groups are treated differently and is clearly measurable. Systemic racism is more complicated, he continued. While there is a lowering of the effect size in each individual part of the system, putting all the parts together—elementary education, high school, college, transitioning, National Institutes of Health (NIH) funding, and more—shows the effect size is large. "That means you have to look at the whole system," he stressed. "What we are really looking for are catalysts that can transform an entire system."

Mr. Gill noted that Doris Duke and other foundations are challenged by implicit bias in allocating resources. He pointed to two features that characterize the role of independent philanthropy as capital allocators. On the one hand, total philanthropic funding is small-scale compared with federal, private, or higher education expenditures. However, he continued, it is also the most independent capital in the world without constraints from investors, public shareholders, or political incentives unless self-imposed. "The theory behind this form of capital is that private wealth aggregation oriented toward the public interest is an important source of innovation and progress," he said.

Related to the first feature about the relative amount of total resources, he related that funding in the science funding community has moved from being catalytic to more incremental, given the high costs of entry to support basic science. Related to the second feature, he continued, "This set of questions—how to build a more inclusive and equitable scientific enterprise—is a phenomenal place for independent capital to be used." Many institutional foundations have adopted commitments to a more equitable enterprise and to dismantling barriers, but, he commented, "we have all done it in our own way; we have become inefficient."

Dr. Parikh described the effort at AAAS to identify barriers. For example, as publisher of *Science*, AAAS is a significant enabler of the scientific enterprise, but the editorial team has historically consisted mostly of white males because hiring practices gave preference to applicants with certain pedigrees. He asked the panelists about other policy changes they have been involved in.

Ms. Davis shared two examples. First, she suggested that health centers look at longstanding policies and practices, often not written down, that have created a more monolithic health system despite the goal of being more place-based. Her organization, which operated 16 hospitals, reexamined human resource policies, such as the language of job descriptions and eligibility requirements, to promote local hiring. As another example, a hospital in the system wanted to plant a vegetable garden to provide fresh food to neighborhood residents receiving government food assistance. This required changing a statute from 1941 that prohibited using government subsidies in small-scale vegetable production. She noted the statute change benefited not just that neighborhood but also other communities across the state. In addition, she pointed out, it was not explicitly a diversity, equity, and inclusion policy, which "shows why it is important to have both traditional and nontraditional partners in the policy space."

Dr. Dzirasa said he spoke from his perspective as a biologist, engineer, and psychiatrist. "It's important to wrestle with why we haven't made changes thus far. We as human beings are a social species, and we have an innate preference toward sameness," he commented. He described a study that showed the acceptance of ideas from so-called in-groups compared with those from out-groups. Using machine learning, doctoral theses written over the past 30 years were analyzed to see how the ideas they contained entered the field. Ideas from the in-group were more likely to have an impact.[1]

Intellect is universally distributed across the population, Dr. Dzirasa stated. "If intellect is universally distributed and not everyone has an opportunity to participate, then it is a suboptimized system," he continued, and policies that bring the best talent forward are essential:

> As the population becomes more diverse and intellect is universally distributed, it means there is less talent over time to be drawing upon. If we care about how this country is going in terms of innovations and treatment, particularly within a global enterprise, we are becoming less fit to do that every single year. The beginning of every policy change is a human question—are we prepared to wrestle with the question, "Do we believe that intellect is universally distributed?"

Mr. Gill commented that "scale is the word of the moment.... But the question is how to use lower investment amounts to trigger larger amounts to be sufficient for transformational change." He said foundations come at scale from two directions: by lowering the transaction costs to adopting a good idea or by changing the level of ambition, for example, through advocacy or building movements. The clarity and urgency of the argument for justice is at a high level and, once the concept of universal distribution of intellect is accepted, there is a huge competitive interest in not leaving talent on the sidelines. The flaw in these arguments, he contended, is the assumption that all the nodes in a system remain static and good ideas are populated across the system. But, he countered, some parts of the system are exacerbating problems, while others are working to solve problems beyond their resources. He suggested doubling the funding that goes to Historically Black Colleges and Universities and math and science initiatives as an effective example of a way to populate the science, technology, engi-

---

[1] For more information, see https://www.pnas.org/doi/10.1073/pnas.1915378117.

neering, and mathematics (STEM) workforce. "We already have a solution at scale that just needs more resources," he said.

Dr. Dzirasa referred to the book *Built to Last* (Collins and Porras, 1994) that urges visionary companies to "try a lot of things and some will work." He noted this approach extends to workforce challenges. Successes have occurred, but there is no systematic way to evaluate what does and does not work. "One of the policy challenges is we need a national system to think about the whole enterprise, figure out what has worked, and scale those things. We need a PI [principal investigator] for that experiment," he suggested.

TRACKING GOOD IDEAS

Mr. Gill said there is an abundance, almost an overabundance, of ideas. He agreed with the idea of a PI-type experiment and a national strategy. It is important to keep what works, not just keep what is already happening, he commented. After rigorous experimentation, he urged investing in the things that work.

Ms. Davis noted that policies set the stage for who has access to funding and opportunities. Who makes the policies is also important. "It's important for funders to look at how decisions are made and if they are being made equitably," she said. Mr. Gill added that funders should be more self-critical. "Philanthropies can be sanctimonious about their mission and values, but less willing to do the hard work," he said, such as looking at how funding evaluation criteria may be unintentionally excluding some populations.

In terms of other concrete changes, Dr. Dzirasa observed that scientific trajectories have changed and most Ph.D.'s are not on academic routes today. A critical need is to promote and share role models of scientific professionals outside of academia, he suggested.

NEXT STEPS

Dr. Parikh noted possibilities related to opportunity, scale, and funding. AAAS is advocating for employee-like benefits for graduate students in NIH and National Science Foundation (NSF) grants and for NIH to make changes in funding decisions. He asked each panelist for other ideas.

Ms. Davis stressed the need for representation and targeted funding to support the hiring and advancement of a diverse STEM faculty. She also noted the need for student debt management and reduction.

Dr. Dzirasa returned to the idea of a PI-type experiment, perhaps set up through the National Science and Technology Council, to establish a national science and technology initiative, an idea that he and colleagues proposed in an April 2021 article in *Science* (Tilghman et al., 2021). Through such an initiative, a 5- to 10-year experiment could be organized with funding streams from NSF, NIH, and other entities, coordinated across administrations.

Mr. Gill noted that the Doris Duke Foundation found caregiving needs are a critical vector for equity among physician-scientists. A pilot project was set up to provide grants for projects at risk because of researchers' caregiving needs. The foundation has also challenged institutional leadership, including university boards and presidents, to consider this to make longer-term progress. "We have to manage against a set of goals as if they are existential because they *are* existential," he said. "If we don't do that, it will be a continued profusion of small steps and incremental progress."

In response to a participant's comment about changes in language and taxonomies, Mr. Gill noted that one of the foundation's major programs is directed at early-career physician-scientists. A program audit found that women and people of color had low participation. Among the steps taken was a change in the language used in describing the award. Although other changes were made, so it is difficult to pinpoint a single factor, he shared that applications and participation increased among underrepresented groups.

Dr. Dzirasa agreed with the need to "meet people where they are." The tendency in talent recruitment is for everyone to look to the same places. "This is why I always go back to the idea that intellect is evenly distributed. If so, your best return is to go to the place where no one else is going. We have set up systems that do not tap talent that exists in certain places," he said.

Roundtable chair Cato Laurencin, Ph.D. (University of Connecticut Health), commented that in talking about diversity and inclusion, the typical programs do not work because they do not address racism adequately. He called for a path that also encompasses diversity, inclusion, antiracism, and learning, for example in NIH funding.

In concluding the first day of the workshop, Dr. Shirley Malcom (AAAS) reflected on the discussions that positioned the Black community as a science community. Housing disparities and other environment assaults counter that sense of community and send the message, "You are not valued, you are not worth investing in," she said. Children either push back on that message or absorb it, she observed. "The issues of financing, belonging, finding peers and a community—that is what we are looking at when we put antiracist vision on policies in place. The issue is how to create a new norm, rooted in diversity, equity, justice, and fairness. We can see the benefits that accrue to a scientific community that is building from the excellence of the talent pool that is out there," she said.

REFERENCES

Collins, J., and J. Porras. 1994. *Built to Last: Successful Habits of Visionary Companies.* New York: Harper Business.

Hofstra, B., V. V. Kulkarni, S. M.-N. Galvez, and D. A. McFarland. 2020. The diversity–innovation paradox in science. *Proceedings of the National Academy of Sciences* Vol. 117, No. 17. https://doi.org/10.1073/pnas.1915378117.

Tilghman, S., B. Alberts, D. Colon-Ramos, K. Dzirasa, J. Kimble, and H. Varmus. 2021. Concrete steps to diversity the scientific workforce. *Science* 372(6538): 133–135.

7

Reality-Based Observations from Those on the Pathway

Highlights from the Presentations

- Advising committees at predominantly white institutions are often not able to name the unique challenges faced by Black students (Ms. Hoggard).
- Student-athletes at elite institutions can gain strength from each other and from their coaches in dealing with disrespect from others on campus (Ms. Hoggard).
- Science provides a sense of wonder—something that should not be forgotten amid the pressures to navigate the environment and succeed (Ms. Harriot).
- In choosing a mentor, it is important to develop a shared understanding about the commitment and expectations (Ms. Harriot).
- Organizations like the Student National Medical Association can provide networking and mentoring opportunities, especially for students who might not have these opportunities at their home institutions (Dr. Felix).
- Communities of color need us. As Dr. Stewart said, we have to be our own protective factors (Dr. Felix).

Planning committee co-chair Evelynn Hammonds, Ph.D. (Harvard University), facilitated a discussion with three scholars who shared their experiences in recognizing their early interest in science, earning their undergraduate degrees, and moving forward in their careers. At the time of the workshop, they were at three different stages: a master's student planning to apply to M.D./Ph.D. programs, Courtney Hoggard (University of Pennsylvania); a doctoral student, Annica Harriot (University of Maryland School of Medicine); and a medical resident specializing in psychiatry, Gabriel Felix, M.D. (Cambridge Health Alliance/Harvard Medical School).

PRE-MED JOURNEY

Ms. Hoggard began by describing her undergraduate experience at Brown University. "What I noted was that advising committees at predominantly white institutions are afraid of naming the unique challenges faced by Black applicants, and it becomes an attempt to whitewash our experience and lived narrative," she said. "On the flip side, when we say we are going to apply to med school or M.D./Ph.D. programs, we don't get support about how we can utilize the power that comes with being young Black people." Assaults can come in many contexts. She related that when she sat down to take the MCAT (Medical College Admission Test), she had to analyze a passage about a Black woman doctor being mistaken for a nurse—"while I was a young Black woman taking one of the most nerve-wracking tests in my life, trying to become a Black woman doctor."

She said what has gotten her through is to look for Black scholars and doctors who have made it. As an M.D./Ph.D. applicant, she said there is "nothing more gut-wrenching than not seeing anyone on M.D./Ph.D. committees that looks like me, on either the student or faculty levels." When she does see a leading Black professional, she said their position seems unattainable because of its rarity. "Black mentors become the guiding directions. I truly don't know what we would do without them," she said.

Reflecting on her early interests, she recalled choosing a doctor's costume one Halloween, which her father used as an opportunity to talk about and encourage her goal. Over time, she realized it was a dream to become the physician that she wished she always had as a patient—a Black woman.

DOCTORAL STUDIES

"I feel privileged as a Ph.D. candidate in STEM [science, technology, engineering, and mathematics] because my experience has been overwhelmingly positive," Ms. Harriot said, but she added, "When I look back, a lot of labor has been involved in making it a positive experience." She said the biggest contributing factor in shaping her career trajectory was discovering the body of literature that exists on mentorship and experiences of Black people, which she learned about through her involvement with #VanguardStem, an online community for women of color in STEM.[1] That knowledge enabled her to choose a mentor and shape the conversations with him about her expectations. She noted her principal investigator (PI) is an older white man who has committed to helping her feel a sense of belonging in her work.

The biggest challenge, Ms. Harriot said, is that the burden of developing positive experiences is placed on young scholars themselves. "This manifests in the imposter syndrome; we talk about 'what can I do to affirm my belonging' rather than talk to peers and colleagues about what they can do to affirm that sense of belonging." The extra labor is placed on her and other scholars of color in addition to the work to obtain a Ph.D., she added.

Ms. Harriot studies skeletal-muscular atrophy and injury in aging, and her personal passion is space flight. She said she feels fortunate because of the sense of wonder she derives from science, and specifically space flight. As a child, when she declared she wanted to be a cardiovascular surgeon and astronaut, her father suggested she study the heart in space, which is now an aspect of her research. She attended a magnet public high school with female Ph.D. science teachers who fostered her interest in science as a career.

A RESIDENT'S EXPERIENCE

As the most senior member of the panel, Dr. Felix related that he had a nontraditional journey into medicine. He took time between undergraduate and medical school, which he commented has been reflected in other discussions throughout the workshop. He said he did not attend a rigorous high school and struggled in college. Meanwhile, he looked around to see majority peers were primed and ready to navigate the pre-med process, and he did not get into medical school the first time he applied. He had no early mentors or coaches, but what made the difference was involvement in the Student National Medical Association (SNMA).[2] The first time he met a Black doctor was in his sophomore year of college at an SNMA conference.

---

[1] For more information about #VanguardSTEM, see https://www.vanguardstem.com.

[2] The Student National Medical Association "is committed to supporting current and future underrepresented minority medical students, addressing the needs of underserved communities, and increasing the number of clinically excellent, culturally competent, and socially conscious physicians." For more information, see http://snma.org.

After college, he worked as a research lab assistant at Howard University, where a co-worker who was a neurology fellow helped him navigate the medical school process. The financial burden was a big challenge, beginning with the cost of applying to medical school.

EXPERIENCE WITH MENTORS

Dr. Hammonds emphasized the panelists' experiences with mentors. Dr. Felix reported that he has several mentors. "It started with me imagining where I saw myself several years down the line," he explained. He said he identified people who were in positions he would like to be in and also would be honest with him. One is the physician he met at the SNMA conference mentioned above. Dr. Felix stressed the value of "getting encouragement from someone who can pour back into you."

Ms. Harriot said her mentors fall into three categories. First is Dr. Jedidah Isler, the first Black woman to earn a Ph.D. in astrophysics from Yale. "Foundational to our relationship is shared identity," Ms. Harriot commented. Dr. Isler has helped her navigate as a Black woman who is often the "only" in a group and suggested ways to put her best foot forward, she related. Second is her PI, who she said has helped shape her as a scientist. He is also open to her perspective in shaping his mentoring style. Third, she finds value in peer-to-peer mentoring, which she characterized as undervalued but incredibly important in STEM fields.

Ms. Hoggard agreed with the value of different types of mentors. She was a student-athlete in college, and her coach remains one of her closest mentors, although she does not have STEM experience. Ms. Hoggard noted that "student-athletes and coaches can have a unique relationship of them telling us when we are wrong, and telling us when to rest and when to activate energy." Her second group of mentors is past teammates who have become doctors, and the third group is two professors in the Department of Africana at Brown who helped her craft her undergraduate study interests.

Dr. Hammonds observed that none of the presenters explicitly mentioned faculty members within their undergraduate major departments. Dr. Felix concurred that he did not have a mentor within his department and had to look elsewhere. "That's one of the major issues when we talk about a lot of undergraduate institutions," he said. "There are not many options, and a lot of legwork has to be done to find them."

Ms. Harriot reported negative experiences as an undergraduate that made her seek mentors outside her institution. Ms. Hoggard described a white male professor who taught a first-year seminar on Health of Hispaniola in which she was the only student of Haitian-Dominican descent. The relationship evolved to the point where she could challenge some of his assumptions, and he became the secondary reader on her undergraduate thesis.

RELATIONSHIPS WITH WHITE STUDENTS

In responding to a question from Dr. Hammonds, Dr. Felix commented on the "pressure to make yourself more palatable in white spaces." It becomes tiring, for example, to listen to stereotypical comments about Black patients or other patients of color and figure out how to address those comments. In summary, he said his experiences with white colleagues have varied, ranging from allies to traumatic, disrespectful interactions.

Ms. Harriot attended a private, conservative Christian, predominantly white institution. "My voice was silenced and dismissed, and that was tough to deal with," she said. "I wanted to push back, less for my voice to be heard but because I felt a responsibility to make my [white] peers aware about other perspectives. It was exhausting." In contrast, at the University of Maryland School of Medicine, where she is a Meyerhoff fellow, she said she is in a diverse environment and in a lab space that champions equity and belonging. Ms. Hoggard commented that being a Black student-athlete at an institution like Brown University is a "recipe for a lot of stereotyping and comments," especially her first year when others on campus assumed she was pursuing a less rigorous path than pre-med. Hearing those comments pushed her white teammates to step in. "They saw it happening and asked me about it, and we would reflect on it," she said. She added that white teammates also receive negative comments as athletes at elite institutions, which caused them to "see themselves for once in a way that we feel all the time and on amplitude levels."

ADVICE TO YOUNGER STUDENTS

Dr. Hammonds asked each scholar to reflect on what they would tell students who are considering the paths that they have chosen and why they should persist.

Ms. Hoggard began. "I would tell them it is going to be hard. I wish someone had been honest with me upfront. I would also tell them there are resources and mentors. Why stay? In my experience, nothing feels more peaceful than knowing that if I stay and plant my feet, that gives someone else another person to look to. The more we stand in our right to be physicians, the more likely there are more of us to stand with us. Plant your feet and don't let someone move you."

Ms. Harriot continued. "To whittle down my feelings, I stay because I matter, and they [younger students] should stay because they do, too. I love science. One of the greatest feelings is when I am in the lab, imaging a new target, and there is a moment when I am doing an experiment before I share the results with my PI where I am the only person who knows the thing I just found. That's amazing. My contributions matter, and the things that only I can do matter—and each one of us has that same capacity."

Dr. Felix added his thoughts. "What I say to students now is, We need you. Our communities need you; they need us. Dr. Stewart put it best: We have to be our own protective factors. In my line of work, one of the most gratifying factors is when I have a patient of color—that look of relief when they see someone who looks like them. We are needed to heal our community. That's one of the reasons we need Black students to stay in STEM."

Dr. Hammonds praised the courage of the panelists in speaking about their personal experiences at a public workshop. "At the same time," she continued, "I would like to have thought in the almost 30 years since I earned my Ph.D., that there would be less of a sense of isolation and less of a need to do so much yourselves. We still have a lot of work to do."

Dr. Pinn asked the presenters for recommendations in overcoming the kinds of psychological barriers discussed at the workshop. Ms. Harriot suggested reevaluating styles and responsibilities of STEM mentorship across such intersections as race and sex, something she has explored with her mentor and written about (Harriot, 2021). Ms. Hoggard noted she is in the medical school cycle, and the labor to find diversity statistics and faculty mentors falls on young people of color. She suggested facilitating this search. Dr. Felix suggested learning how to set healthy boundaries for mentees and mentors, and communicate expectations clearly. "It's important to protect our mental health while we help to cultivate the future," he said.

REFERENCE

Harriot, A. 2021. A practical guide to mentoring across intersections. *VanguardSTEM Conversations*. https://conversations.vanguardstem.com/a-practical-guide-to-mentoring-across-intersections-c596496ee334.

8

Moving Forward with Urgency

Highlights from the Presentations

- No matter the level of seniority and expertise, Black professionals often encounter the same problems of isolation and being underestimated faced earlier in their careers, but they have learned how to handle them (Dr. Malcom).
- The same problems faced by Black students and young professionals 30 years ago persist today (Dr. Hammonds).
- As demographics, the scientific workforce, and mentality about ourselves have changed, the system needs to change to accommodate us, not us having to change to fit in (Dr. Pinn).
- It is okay to say I am not okay. Whether we are talking about the high school student with an interest in STEM or the practicing physician or the more seasoned clinician, there should not be a stigma in accessing mental wellness services (Dr. Stewart).

The workshop was structured to include informal discussion among the committee co-chairs in a fireside chat format, followed by opening the conversation to other presenters and participants. It closed with a keynote by Roundtable member Cora Marrett, Ph.D. (University of Wisconsin–Madison).

"FIRESIDE CHAT": DR. VIVIAN PINN, DR. SHIRLEY MALCOM, DR. ALTHA STEWART, AND DR. EVELYNN HAMMONDS

Dr. Pinn opened the session by noting that when she, Dr. Malcom, and Dr. Hammonds tapped into the literature to plan the workshop, they found the research on the need to build resilience early in life particularly striking. She also commented that the frequent conversations they held as co-chairs reinforced their bonds. Dr. Malcom reflected on the importance of "checking in with each other" at all stages of life. She continued:

> What is important—no matter how old you get, how far you go, how distinguished the awards you get, we still encounter the same problems we had earlier in our careers. We face many of the same problems, in terms of isolation, in terms of low expectations from others. I just learned how to handle them differently.

Keynote presenter Dr. Stewart (see Chapter 2) responded to Dr. Malcom's comments. She stressed the value of conversations around wellness. "I really want us to shift our language so that being well is the natural state," she said. She agreed with Dr. Malcom's observation about facing low expectations and being underestimated by the majority community. "I enjoy that look on people's faces when they realize that I am present, I am all there," she said. This is part of her cultural wealth, she said. "I have to point out to people that not recognizing that in me is their problem." She noted she continues to honor and emulate role models, and she stressed the responsibility that she and others have to shepherd and protect younger professionals. Dr. Hammonds observed that many issues young people are dealing with today, such as how to navigate the system, have persisted for years. Despite the presence of many programs and resources, she said, "I don't understand why we still can't get this information to the people who need it. Where are we failing our younger people?" She urged development of a repository of information to facilitate access, to which Dr. Stewart added the need for an accountability structure.

Dr. Malcom suggested that actions to assist early-career scientists could include a requirement that National Institutes of Health (NIH) funding require the existence of a mentoring compact between a mentor and mentee, one of the tools for effective mentoring suggested by a recent National Academies of Sciences, Engineering, and Medicine committee.[1] Another issue to hammer out, she continued, relates to graduate students receiving appropriate credit as co-authors in papers or co-inventors in patents. These are rules that graduate students must learn and work out ahead of time, and they need guidance in knowing them.

Referring to Ms. Harriot's conversations with her principal investigator (PI; see Chapter 7), Dr. Hammonds stressed the importance of faculty and students setting expectations in a supportive way. Students should not have to be fortunate enough to "fall into" helpful situations, she said. "The problem to me is building the capacity and holding accountable the people who are in charge of educating students in STEM [science, technology, engineering, and mathematics]," she stated.

The default, Dr. Stewart observed, is for those in power to help those who are like them. "If I am not like you, I do not come to your attention when it comes to decisions about who gets into a program, who you go looking for to recruit into the program," she commented. "We are not the natural thinking point." She suggested the NIH UNITE program (see Chapter 5) may open the door by tying the need for more inclusive recruitment and working climates into the distribution of funds.

"We have to remember that we did not create these spaces," observed Dr. Malcom. "They were created by people for their lives and experiences. And that's okay—but do not put barriers in my way." In a recent presentation to the National Science Board, she emphasized not just the quality of research but also the quality of the research environment, because "you will not get a good return on investment in an environment of exclusion."[2] These comments touch on the theme of the workshop, observed Dr. Pinn. "As demographics, the scientific workforce, and our mentality about ourselves have changed, the system needs to change to accommodate us, not us having to change to fit in," she said. She pointed to SEA Change, the program that Dr. Malcom directs at the American Association for the Advancement of Science, which provides a systems look and accountability structure.[3]

Dr. Hammonds returned to Ms. Harriot's comment about approaching science with a sense of wonder (see Chapter 7). The sense of wonder

---

[1] For more information on this and other tools, see "The Science of Effective Mentoring in STEMM," https://www.nationalacademies.org/our-work/the-science-of-effective-mentoring-in-stemm.

[2] A recording of her August 10, 2021, presentation may be seen on the National Science Board's YouTube channel at https://www.youtube.com/watch?v=nbIFM0KHEao.

[3] For more information about SEA Change, see https://seachange.aaas.org.

that draws young people to science should not be lost in the struggle to get through the system, she said. Dr. Pinn urged following through with ideas that have brought success, rather than continuing to "spend years talking about where we need to go." Dr. Stewart agreed models exist that are ready to go to scale. She urged funders to come together to make long-term commitments to support programs that start in middle school. The commitment, she continued, must establish metrics and outcomes with the end goal to increase the pool of trained, culturally responsive professionals.

TOWN HALL

To open up to a town-hall format, Dr. Pinn first asked Dr. Stewart to reflect on what she heard during the workshop since setting the stage with her opening keynote (see Chapter 2). Dr. Stewart began by stressing:

> It is okay to say I am not okay. Let's start there. Whether we are talking about the high school student with an interest in STEM or the practicing physician or the more seasoned clinician—at every stage of life. It is particularly important to say that out loud in communities of color because we are so tuned into stigma and discrimination and the assumption that we are not up to the task. It is critical to set aside that myth, because people are not seeking out the services they need.

She continued that if young professionals are having the same experiences that more senior professional had years ago, "We have no choice. It is our fundamental responsibility to say, 'no more' and to make a difference. The reality is we can muster the psychological strength with the support of others. The reality is that racism does exist, and people do not want us to succeed in large numbers."

There are solutions, she continued. A workshop like this can bring together those with lived experience and the content expertise to craft blueprints for action. "We are the solution we have been waiting for. We are the right people to put this in front of the right person, agency, or organization," Dr. Stewart said.

Kenneth Hill, reflecting on his experience setting up programs in Detroit and Chicago (see Chapter 3), said he crystallizes his thoughts into three sentences: "First, our children are brilliant. Second, our parents want their children to do well. Third, if we can get together to help our parents help their children excel at early age, in my opinion that is the key."

Roundtable member Lynne Holden, M.D. (Albert Einstein College of Medicine), shared four lessons that she has learned through Mentoring in Medicine, the nonprofit organization she leads that has helped 500 students get into and through medical school. First, listen to the students, parents, and educators to learn their needs and perceived obstacles. Second, start young to teach children to ask questions and nurture their intellectual curiosity. Third, provide supplemental help through after-school and other programs. Fourth, embed social and emotional intelligence in programming so students can deal with implicit bias, imposter syndrome, and other challenges.

Several comments centered on the value of early intervention. Roundtable member Charles Bridges, M.D., Ph.D. (Janssen Pharmaceuticals), commented on what he has learned through involvement in a Philadelphia math and reading enrichment program.[4] With appropriate resources, a group of 25 Black public school students in grades 3 and 4 who had below-grade math and reading scores were at or above grade level within several years. Mr. Hill reported that the W. K. Kellogg Foundation is funding development of an algebra concepts program for K–3 in which parents and children learn side by side. Ms. Harriot commented that she was shaped to become a scientist through STEM magnet programs in middle and high school.

Dr. Felix recommended advocating to ensure faculty of color are supported as they serve as mentors. Many are the only person of color in their department or organization, and they are at capacity. Dr. Pinn concurred with the challenge for faculty of color who are asked to serve on multiple committees while also trying to do their own research. She acknowledged the debate over this issue. She said for her, committee involvement increased her exposure and "got me to the table." Dr. Malcom said tenure and promotion criteria must be addressed so that faculty are not just judged by the number of grants and publications, but how they are teaching, mentoring, and coaching diverse student populations.

In response to a question Dr. Hammonds asked about increasing the numbers of African Americans working in mental health fields, Dr. Stewart reiterated her call for the breaking down of stigma barriers, as well as ensuring the field is in tune with what is beneficial to Black people. She suggested

---

[4] See Kumon Math and Reading Program, available at https://www.kumon.com/.

three strategies. First, the Black Psychiatrists of America and other groups should outline strategies to reach out to students in the early stages of medical training to consider specializing in psychiatry. Second, psychiatric training programs and residencies must have diversity, equity, and inclusion (DEI) as a priority. Third, agencies such as the Substance Abuse and Mental Health Services Administration and the National Institute of Mental Health should support long-term training plans to grow the workforce to meet their diversity targets.

Roundtable member Gilda Barabino, Ph.D. (Olin College of Engineering), commented that the discussion reflects the challenges that Black STEM professionals face, no matter their position on the career ladder. She emphasized the need to start early and stay with students throughout their entire pathway. "The time is now—and it is the time for us to take ownership and not wait for someone else to do it," she said.

CLOSING KEYNOTE

Dr. Marrett reflected on the presentations and participants' comments, noting the emphasis on how to put into action what was shared. She also shared the question from one participant who asked "if we are preaching to the choir." Dr. Marrett responded, "Yes, but what's wrong with that? What's wrong with trying to strengthen voices and enhance harmony if we want to have a choir to sing in ways that others are going to hear." Returning to the "singing of the choir" analogy during her remarks, she reviewed what she saw as takeaways throughout the workshop.

She echoed Dr. Altha Stewart's call for protective factors to help navigate challenges in moving forward. "We must provide our own protective veneer," Dr. Marrett stressed.

She also observed that the explanations given for limited participation by persons of color in STEM have changed over time. Inequities are no longer attributed, at least publicly, to limits in African Americans' abilities and talents. A more prevailing view, often implicit, is that the reasons for underrepresentation lie within the targeted communities. Presentations from the workshop dispute this view, she pointed out. Dr. Kevin Cokley and Dr. Sonya Douglass Horsford (see Chapters 2 and 3) discredited the argument that curiosity and willingness to work hard are absent from targeted communities. Further evidence from Mr. Hill and others (see Chapter 3) point to strong parental support for children's achievements and learning. And Dr. Ebony McGee (see Chapter 2) described the pursuit by many graduate students to achieve in STEM fields despite being under financial and psychological stress. In summary, she stated, "A number of the assumptions about what is lacking do not hold up under close scrutiny. That is an issue that is important for the Roundtable and for whom we interact with."

Dr. Marrett noted support by many participants for Dr. Gordon's statement that the Black community must create conditions to foster young people's achievements (see Chapter 3). However, she cautioned that models and strategies must be appropriate for given circumstances. For example, the concept of mentoring is universally endorsed, she observed, but mentoring models are often taken off the shelf and do not reflect the experiences and needs that can exist. She called attention to successes at the University of Maryland, Baltimore County and Morehouse School of Medicine, among others (see Chapter 4).

Several speakers raised the question of resistance to change, Dr. Marrett pointed out. When resources are expanding, she observed, diversity initiatives are generally supported. However, she said, "when there are limits on the resources, we see very different kinds of approaches. We see resistance." Further, she said, the concepts of diversity, equity, and inclusion often are "thrown together," but they have different outcomes. "Diversity—having numbers based on representation in the population—is not the same as inclusion, with full engagement and participation," she said. Quoting a workshop participant, Dr. Marrett said, "The DEI lens needs to be agreed upon. There are so many models that it makes measurement difficult and makes the pursuit extremely difficult." It takes more than the existence of a DEI plan.

A multitude of reports start with statements that diversity is important for the nation and the world, Dr. Marrett said, but sometimes these are just words. Instead, she said, "if we believe deeply that the advances and future of the nation depends on how well we use all our resources, how well we reach out to the talent that is there, if that is what we have in mind, then we need to stand behind how this is more than words, more than a mission or vision statement." She continued:

> There is comfort in knowing that one is not addressing these problems and issues alone. It can be so easy to feel isolated, and that is not a comforting matter. Engagement with others seems especially important when we are talking about systemic issues. These are not issues that can be easily handled by individuals. It's

> the kind of collective involvement and sense you can derive from having people on the same page—singing from the same hymnal.

Dr. Marrett noted the workshop co-chairs have been attuned to how to use the knowledge, for whom and for what. She concluded by "thanking the choir" for their music, harmonies, and willingness to think about how to get other ears to understand, hear, and interact.

CONCLUDING REMARKS BY THE WORKSHOP CO-CHAIRS

Dr. Malcom reiterated the message from Dr. Marrett that "if we are going to make system-level change, we cannot do it alone. Essentially it is a collective effort, not an individual one." Dr. Hammonds said she felt a sense of transformation from the workshop discussions. Dr. Pinn thanked committee members, participants, and the National Academies staff. "We need to keep thinking about moving forward and preserving mental wellness for all of us, especially for the next generation so [that] they inherit a world in which they can be successful and further the excitement of the science that they will be taking over from us as we move on."

Appendix A

Workshop Agenda

DAY ONE
SEPTEMBER 14, 2021 – 9:30 AM – 5:15 PM EST

9:30 – 10:00 AM ET **Opening Remarks and Introductions:**

Dr. Laura Castillo-Page, Ph.D.
Chief Diversity and Inclusion Officer, the National Academies of Sciences, Engineering, and Medicine

Dr. Cato T. Laurencin, M.D., Ph.D.
Chair of the Roundtable

Dr. Vivian W. Pinn, M.D., Co-chair
Dr. Shirley Malcom, Ph.D., Co-chair
Dr. Evelynn Hammonds, Ph.D., Co-chair

SESSION I: ADDRESSING MENTAL HEALTH AND SOCIO-PSYCHOLOGICAL FACTORS TO INCREASE THE PARTICIPATION OF BLACK WOMEN AND MEN IN SEM

10:00 – 10:15 AM **Opening Keynote:**

Dr. Altha J. Stewart, Associate Professor of Psychiatry and Director, Center for Health in Justice Involved Youth, University of Tennessee Health Science Center; First Black President of the American Psychiatric Association; Past President of the Association of Women Psychiatrists and Past President of the Black Psychiatrists of America

Introduction by: **Dr. Vivian W. Pinn**, Senior Scientist Emerita, Fogarty International Center, NIH, Founding Director, Office of Research on Women's Health, NIH (Retired)

10:15 – 11:00 AM **The Importance of the Mission: Setting the Stage for Change**

Moderator & Presenter: **Dr. Kevin Cokley**, Chair, Department of Educational Psychology; University and UT System Distinguished Teaching Professor, Oscar and Anne Mauzy Regents Professor for Educational Research and Development, Professor of Educational Psychology and African and African Diaspora Studies, University of Texas at Austin

Panelist: **Dr. Ebony O. McGee**, Professor of Education, Diversity and STEM (Science, Technology, Engineering, & Mathematics) Education, Department of Teaching and Learning, Vanderbilt University's Peabody College

Responder: **Dr. Thomas Vance**, Visiting Research Scholar, The New School

11:00 – 11:15 AM Discussion and Q & A

SESSION II: EARLY EDUCATION AS THE PATHWAY TO SUCCESS: PRE-K TO 12

11:15 – 11:40 AM **Pre-K–12 as Foundational for Future in SEM**

Moderator: **Dr. Shirley Malcom**, Head of Education and Human Resources Programs of the American Association for the Advancement of Science

Presenter: **Dr. Edmund W. Gordon**, John M. Musser Professor of Psychology, Emeritus, Yale University, Richard March Hoe Professor, Emeritus of Psychology and Education, Founding Director of the Institute of Urban and Minority Education, Teachers College, Columbia University

Presenter: **Kenneth Hill**, President and CEO ChiS&E

11:40 AM – 12:30 PM **Panel Discussion**

Panelists:

- **Dr. Jean-Claude Brizard**, President and CEO, Digital Promise
- **Dr. Bernard Harris, M.D.**, CEO, National Math-Science Initiative (NMSI)
- **Dr. Sonya Douglass Horsford**, Professor and Founding Director, Black Education Research Collective (BERC), Teachers College, Columbia University

Responder: **Dr. Edmund W. Gordon**

12:30 – 12:45 PM Discussion and Q & A

12:45 PM – 1:15 PM Break for Lunch

SESSION III: HIGHER EDUCATION AND INSTITUTIONAL CHANGES

1:15 PM – 2:15 PM **Changes at Colleges and Universities to Assure Access, Success, and Well-Being**

Moderator: **Dr. Evelynn Hammonds**, Barbara Gutmann Rosenkrantz Professor of the History of Science; Professor of African and African American Studies; Chair, Department of the History of Science; Director, Project on Race & Gender in Science & Medicine, Hutchins Center for African and African American Research, Harvard University

Presenters:

- **Dr. Valerie Montgomery Rice, M.D.**, President, Morehouse School of Medicine
- **Dr. Keivan Stassun, Ph.D.**, Stevenson Prof. of Astrophysics, College of Arts and Sciences, Prof. of Computer Science, Vanderbilt School of Engineering, Director, Frist Autism and Innovation at Vanderbilt, and Adjunct Prof. of Physics, Fisk University
- **Dr. Mike Summers, Ph.D.**, Professor of Chemistry, UMBC
- **Dr. Kimberly M. Jackson, Ph.D.**, Professor and Chair Department of Chemistry, Spelman College; Co-director of the living and learning community for STEM scholars

2:15 – 2:30 PM Discussion and Q & A

SESSION IV: BRINGING SYSTEMIC CHANGES THROUGH IMPORTANT SECTORS OF INFLUENCE

2:30 – 3:30 PM **Opportunities to Support a More Systemic Approach to Addressing Mental and Behavioral Health**

Moderator: **Dr. Garth Graham, M.D., M.P.H., F.A.C.P., F.A.C.C.**, Director and Global Head of Healthcare and Public Health Google and Head of YouTube Health

Presenters:
- **Dr. Laurie Zephyrin, M.D., M.P.H., M.B.A.**, Vice President for Advancing Health Equity at the Commonwealth Fund Boule
- **Dr. Marie Bernard**, Chief Officer for Scientific Workforce Diversity, NIH
- **Dr. Cora B. Marrett**, Former Deputy Director, National Science Foundation
- **Dr. Nwando Olayiwola M.D., M.P.H.**, Chief Health Equity Officer & Senior Vice President, Humana

3:30 – 3:45 PM Discussion and Q & A

SESSION V: DEVELOPMENT AND IMPLEMENTATION OF EQUITY-BASED STRATEGIES

3:45 – 5:00 PM **Coordinated Responses across Agencies, Organizations, and Departments to Address Disparities and Barriers**

Moderator: **Dr. Sudip Parikh**, CEO, AAAS

Panelists:
- **Dr. Kafui Dzirasa**, Associate Professor of Psychiatry and Behavioral Science, Duke University

- **Michellene Davis, Esq.**, President and CEO, National Medical Fellowships, Inc.
- **Samsher Singh Gill**, President and CEO, Doris Duke Charitable Foundation

4:45 – 5:00 PM Discussion and Q&A

5:00 – 5:15 PM **Discussion, Wrap-up, and Next Steps by Workshop Co-Chairs**

5:15 PM **Day One Adjourned**

DAY TWO
SEPTEMBER 15, 2021 – 1:15 – 5:00 PM EST

SESSION VI: SOLUTIONS THAT RESULT IN SYSTEMIC CHANGES: GATEWAYS AND GATEKEEPERS

1:15 – 2:15 PM **Panel for Reality-Based Observations from Those in the Pathway**

Moderator: **Evelynn Hammonds**

Panelists:

- **Courtney Hoggard**, Master of Bioethics candidate at University of Pennsylvania, and recent pre-med student, Brown University
- **Anicca Harriot, Ph.D.**, student in the Graduate Program in Life Sciences, Biochemistry and Molecular Biology Program and Meyerhoff Graduate Fellows Program at the University of Maryland School of Medicine.
- **Dr. Gabriel Felix, M.D.**, Psychiatry Resident at Cambridge Health Alliance/Harvard Medical School.

2:00 PM – 2:15 PM Discussion and Q & A

2:15 – 3:00 PM **Fireside chat** – Co-Chairs and Committee will reflect on questions such as:

- Why are mental health considerations vital for systemic changes?
- What are the actions that are needed to move forward after today?
- Which sectors of influence, from educational components, to government, communities, the scientific community, and even families, need to be involved?

3:00 – 4:00 PM **Audience Town Hall Discussion** on Innovative Strategies Required for Systemic Changes to Pave a Smooth Pathway for Black Men and Women into Successful Careers in Science, Engineering, and Medicine

SESSION VII: MOVING FORWARD WITH URGENCY – CLOSING KEYNOTE ADDRESS

4:00 – 4:45 PM **Closing Keynote speaker: Dr. Cora Marrett**

Moderator: **Dr. Vivian Pinn**

4:45 – 5:00 PM **Closing comments and pathways for action from the Co-Chairs**

5:00 PM **Day Two and Workshop Adjourns**

Appendix B

Biographical Sketches of Presenters

SPEAKERS

Marie A. Bernard is the National Institutes of Health (NIH) chief officer for scientific workforce diversity (COSWD). As COSWD, she leads NIH's science of scientific workforce diversity, building, disseminating, and acting on the evidence. Her office is the NIH thought leader in assuring optimal scientific creativity and innovation, both intramurally and extramurally, through a diverse scientific workforce. Dr. Bernard also co-leads NIH's UNITE initiative to end structural racism. Prior to being selected as the COSWD in May 2021, she was deputy director of the National Institute on Aging (2008–2021). As an academic geriatrician, she has been recognized widely for leadership in geriatrics research, teaching, and clinical practice. Her work within NIH has been recognized with NIH Director's Awards (2018 and 2019), including the 2020 NIH Director's Award for Equity, Diversity, and Inclusion.

Jean-Claude Brizard is president and CEO of Digital Promise, a global, nonpartisan, nonprofit organization focused on accelerating innovation in education. He is former senior advisor and deputy director in U.S. Programs at the Bill and Melinda Gates Foundation where he focused on PK–16 education across five communities in four states. He also led several strategies to help close the racial and economic achievement gaps in

Washington State's educational system as well as to support the growth and sustainability of the state's public charter school sector.

He is the former chief executive of Chicago Public Schools. Prior to his appointment in Chicago, he was superintendent of schools for the Rochester, New York, School District. Under Mr. Brizard's leadership, both the Chicago Public Schools and the Rochester City School District saw substantial improvements in student performance. Mr. Brizard's experience also includes a 21-year career as an educator and administrator with the NYC Department of Education. He served as a regional superintendent, supervising more than 100 schools in the Borough of Brooklyn and he also served as the system's executive director for its 400 secondary schools. He is a fellow of the Broad Center, a fellow of the Pahara-Aspen Institute, and a member of the Aspen Institute Global Leadership Network.

Laura Castillo-Page is chief diversity and inclusion officer at the National Academies of Sciences, Engineering, and Medicine, where she leads the development of an overall diversity, equity, and inclusion (DEI) strategy and set of programs for the entire organization. Prior to coming to the National Academies, Dr. Castillo-Page most recently served as senior director for equity, diversity, and inclusion at the Association of American Medical Colleges (AAMC). She holds a Ph.D. and M.S. in educational administration and policy studies as well as an M.A. in political science from the University at Albany, SUNY, and holds a B.A. in political science and Latin American studies from Fordham University.

Kafui Dzirasa completed a Ph.D. in neurobiology at Duke University. His research interests focus on understanding how changes in the brain produce neurological and mental illness, and his graduate work has led to several distinctions including the Somjen Award for Most Outstanding Dissertation Thesis, the Ruth K. Broad Biomedical Research Fellowship, the UNCF·Merck Graduate Science Research Fellowship, and the Wakeman Fellowship. Dr. Dzirasa obtained an M.D. from the Duke University School of Medicine in 2009, and he completed residency training in general psychiatry in 2016.

Dr. Dzirasa received the Charles Johnson Leadership Award in 2007, and he was recognized as one of *Ebony* magazine's 30 Young Leaders of the Future in February 2008. He has also been awarded the International Mental Health Research Organization Rising Star Award and the Sydney Baer Prize for Schizophrenia Research, and his laboratory was featured on

CBS 60 Minutes in 2011. In 2016, he was awarded the inaugural Duke Medical Alumni Emerging Leader Award and the Presidential Early Career Award for Scientists and Engineers, the nation's highest award for scientists and engineers in the early stages of their independent research careers. In 2017, he was recognized as 40 under 40 in Health by the National Minority Quality Forum, and the Engineering Alumni of the Year from the University of Maryland, Baltimore County. He was induced into the American Society for Clinical Investigation in 2019.

Dr. Dzirasa has served as an associate scientific advisor for the journal *Science Translational Medicine*, as a member of the congressionally mandated Next Generation Research Initiative, on the Editorial Advisory Board for TEDMED, and on the NIH Director's guiding committee for the BRAIN Initiative. He currently serves on the NIH Director's Novel and Exceptional Technology and Research Advisory Committee (NExTRAC) and Brain Multi-Council Working Group.

Dr. Dzirasa is an associate professor at Duke University with appointments in the Departments of Psychiatry and Behavioral Sciences, Neurobiology, Biomedical Engineering, and Neurosurgery. His ultimate goal is to combine his research, medical training, and community experience to improve outcomes for diverse communities suffering from neurological and psychiatric illness.

Gabriel Felix is a physician completing adult psychiatry training at Cambridge Health Alliance (CHA)/Harvard Medical School (HMS). He received his medical degree from Howard University College of Medicine. While in medical school, he held multiple positions of leadership at local and national levels, including serving as the 55th national president for the Student National Medical Association (SNMA) and as an officer on the Board of Trustees of the National Medical Association (NMA). His nonclinical skill set includes event planning, developing programmatic agendas, strategic planning, and public speaking. He is an active member in several professional organizations, including the NMA, the American Psychiatric Association (APA), the American Medical Association (AMA), and the Black Psychiatrists of America (BPA), among others. He is currently a Public Psychiatry fellow for the American Psychiatric Association and serves as the postgraduate physician trustee for the National Medical Association. He continues his involvement in the SNMA as a mentor for premedical and medical students.

Samsher (Sam) Singh Gill is the third president and CEO of the Doris Duke Charitable Foundation (DDCF), a New York-headquartered, national philanthropic organization that supports the performing arts, medical research, the environment, and child well-being. He also serves as president of several operating foundations that run under DDCF's umbrella, including the Duke Farms Foundation, which operates a center for environmental stewardship in Hillsborough, New Jersey, and the Doris Duke Foundation for Islamic Art, which operates a museum for learning about the global cultures of Islamic art and design in Honolulu, Hawai'i, as well as a New York-based grants program with a related mission.

Prior to joining DDCF in April 2021, Mr. Gill was senior vice president and chief program officer at the John S. and James L. Knight Foundation, where he oversaw more than $100 million in annual grant making across the foundation's programs, in addition to managing Knight's research and assessment portfolio and its grants administration function. Previously, he also served as vice president of Freedman Consulting, LLC.

Mr. Gill also served on the board of the Philip and Patricia Frost Museum of Science in Miami and on the Commission on the Practice of Democratic Citizenship, a project of the American Academy of Arts and Sciences. He attended the University of Chicago and the University of Oxford, where he was a Rhodes Scholar.

Edmund W. Gordon is the director emeritus of the Institute for Urban and Minority Education at Teachers College of Columbia University. He is also John M. Musser Professor of Psychology, Emeritus, at Yale University and the Richard March Hoe Professor, Emeritus of Psychology and Education at Teachers College of Columbia University. He has served as a senior scholar in residence for the College Board since 1993, and was the chairperson of the Gordon Commission on the Future of Assessment for the Educational Testing Service from 2011 to 2013. He is a fellow of the American Academy of Science and Humanities, the American Association for the Advancement of Science, the American Psychological Society, the American Psychological Association, and the Educational Testing Service and holds honorary degrees from several universities, including Howard University, Mount Holyoke College, Brown University, and Yale University. Dr. Gordon has published extensively on education, justice, and the hidden curriculum.

Anicca Harriot is a biochemistry and molecular biology Ph.D. candidate at the University of Maryland School of Medicine. Her research focuses on the mechanisms responsible for skeletal muscle atrophy and injury. Ms. Harriot plans to use her degree to explore the effects of long-duration space missions on the human body and hopes to someday venture out into the final frontier for herself. She also serves as the chief of community development for #VanguardSTEM: Conversations for Women of Color in STEM, a nonprofit dedicated to lifting the voices of women and nonbinary people of color in STEM. Through #VanguardSTEM, she is able to deploy her passion for advocacy and science communication alongside other women of color and nonbinary people of color in STEM to self-advocate by fully representing themselves and their STEM identities and interests, without assimilation. Ms. Harriot's passion for advocacy and prominent influence has led her to being recognized as one of Motherboard's 2017 Humans of the Year, a 2017 Young Futurist for The Root, and most recently as a 2020 President's Fellow at the University of Maryland, Baltimore.

Bernard Harris is CEO of the National Math and Science Initiative and leads the organization's efforts to improve teacher effectiveness and student achievement in communities across the country. He has been involved in math and science education for over 25 years through his philanthropy as founder of the Harris Institute/Foundation. He also served as managing partner of Vesalius Ventures, Inc., a venture capital firm that invests in early- to mid-stage health-care technologies and companies. He is responsible for managing a portfolio of private assets of early- and mid- stage venture investments and operating companies.

Dr. Harris was at NASA for 10 years, where he conducted research in musculoskeletal physiology and clinical investigations of space adaptation and developed in-flight medical devices to extend astronaut stays in space. A veteran astronaut for over 20 years, he has logged more than 438 hours and traveled over 7.2 million miles in space.

He is a member of the Board of Directors for U.S. Physical Therapy, Raytheon Technologies (RTX), and Monebo Technologies. Dr. Harris serves as a board of director/trustee for Salient Midstream & MLP Fund and Salient MF Trust, and Barings Fund & Trust. In addition, he serves on the National Academies of Sciences, Engineering, and Medicine's Board on Health Sciences Policy, the Texas Medical Center, the National Math and Science Initiative, and the Harris Institute/Foundation.

He earned a bachelor of science in biology from the University of Houston, a master of medical science from the University of Texas Medical Branch at Galveston, a master of business administration from the University of Houston, and a doctorate of medicine from Texas Tech University School of Medicine. He completed a residency in internal medicine at the Mayo Clinic, a National Research Council Fellowship in Endocrinology at the NASA Ames Research Center, and trained as a flight surgeon at the Aerospace School of Medicine, Brooks Air Force Base. He is also a licensed private pilot and certified scuba diver.

Dr. Harris is the recipient of numerous awards, including nine honorary doctorates (from Stony Brook University (SUNY), Morehouse School of Medicine, New Jersey Institute of Technology (NJIT), Washington & Jefferson College, Worcester Polytechnic Institute, University of Hartford, Indiana Institute of Technology, University of Houston, and University of the Sciences), the NASA Space Flight Medal and the NASA Award of Merit, and is a fellow of the American College of Physicians; he was the recipient of the 2000 Horatio Alger Award.

Dr. Harris is the author of *Dream Walker: A Journey of Achievement and Inspiration*.

Kenneth Hill has served as the president and CEO of Chicago Pre-College Science and Engineering Program since 2008. He has been recognized throughout his career for curricular innovations, including the founding in 1976, of an award-winning out-of-school urban K–12 (initially middle school) STEM education program—the Detroit Area Pre-College Engineering Program—often cited as a model in its field. He launched Chicago's first K–3 out of school science and engineering program, the Chicago Pre-College Science and Engineering Program (ChiS&E) with support from the National Science Foundation in 2009, which has since expanded to a K–12 program and incorporated pre-algebraic concepts into ChiS&E's K–3 programs, for both students and parents, with support from the W. K. Kellogg Foundation. He holds degrees in civil engineering from Howard University and mathematics education from Wayne State University.

Courtney L. Savage Hoggard is a 2019 graduate of Brown University, where the former student-athlete received a bachelor of arts in health and human biology and Latin American and Caribbean studies. While at Brown, Ms. Hoggard researched post-traumatic stress disorder (PTSD) in a post-disaster state of Tegucigalpa, Honduras, and the role of the American public housing infrastructure and systemic racism on Asthma's categorization as the "Black and Puerto Rican Disease." Since graduating from Brown University, she has worked as an associate at the Milken

Institute in Washington, D.C., and interned at the Commonwealth Fund in New York City, helping to develop the growing vulnerable populations and maternal health body of work under Dr. Laurie Zephyrin. Beginning in the fall of 2021, she enrolled in the master of bioethics program at the University of Pennsylvania. She intends to focus her scholarly project on how systemic racism informs patient autonomy and clinical ethics, further asking how community-oriented primary care can aid in addressing these questions. During this year, Ms. Hoggard is also applying to medical school to continue studying how the history of medicine and science play a role in the upholding of white supremacy within health-care systems.

Sonya Douglass Horsford serves as professor of education leadership at Teachers College, Columbia University, where she conducts research and teaches courses on the politics of race and inequality in education. She has published more than 20 articles in journals such as *Educational Administration Quarterly*, *Education Policy*, and *Teachers College Record*, edited three books on educational equity and leadership, and authored two award-winning books: *Learning in a Burning House: Educational Inequality, Ideology, and (Dis)Integration* and *The Politics of Education Policy in an Era of Inequality: Possibilities for Democratic Schooling* with Janelle T. Scott and Gary L. Anderson.

Since 2016, Dr. Horsford has served as co-director of the Urban Education Leaders Program (UELP) at Teachers College, an Ed.D. program for practicing and aspiring district-level education leaders committed to equity, justice, and excellence. In 2017, Dr. Horsford founded the Black Education Research Collective to convene scholars devoted to conducting, translating, and disseminating research that leads to improved educational opportunities, experiences, and outcomes for Black children and youth. In 2020, she launched the SDH Collaborative (affectionately known as "the Lab") to create a generative and supportive research and learning environment for current and former students interested in solving educational problems through research, advocacy, and action.

Dr. Horsford chairs the Leadership for Social Justice SIG and Politics of Education SIG for the American Educational Research Association (AERA) and serves as TC's Plenum Session Representative to the University Council for Educational Administration (UCEA). She also serves on the advisory boards of Columbia Journalism School's Spencer Fellows Board and Teachers College Press.

Kimberly M. Jackson is chair and professor of chemistry and biochemistry and director of the Food Studies program at Spelman College in Atlanta, Georgia. She is also co-director of a living and learning community for STEM scholars (The LINCS), an initiative whose goal is to improve access to STEM research careers for women of color through professional and social networks and social justice empowerment, while addressing a critical national need by cultivating talent for the STEM workforce. Author of *Realigning the Crooked Room: Spelman Claims a Space for African American Women in STEM,*" Dr. Jackson has mentored more than 40 research students, providing them with research experiences in cancer therapeutics and drug discovery.

As a Fulbright scholar, a visiting faculty at Harvard Medical School, and a research fellow at the Women's International Study Center in Santa Fe, New Mexico, her robust and active research program focuses on novel therapeutic agents for hormone refractory prostate cancer and the role of minority-serving institutions and women of color in diversifying the STEM pipeline; each with a host of publications, presentations, and funding from multiple agencies. She has received the Spelman Presidential Award for Excellence in Research, Teaching, and Mentoring, American Association for Cancer Research MSI Faculty Scholar Award, and the Governor's Teaching Award for her commitment to STEM excellence. She serves on the national advisory board for COACh for Women Scientists, the American Chemical Society Committee on Minority Affairs, and the American Society of Biochemistry and Molecular Biology Public Affairs program with the goal of helping advocate for and implement policies to promote best practices for recruitment, retention, career development, and evaluation of programs for the advancement of Black women scientists.

Cato Laurencin is the eighth designated University Professor in the 135 year history of the University of Connecticut. He is the Albert and Wilda Van Dusen Distinguished Endowed Professor of Orthopaedic Surgery. He is the CEO of the Connecticut Convergence Institute for Translation in Regenerative Engineering and the director of the Raymond and Beverly Sackler Center for Biomedical, Biological, Physical and Engineering Sciences at the University of Connecticut. Dr. Laurencin earned a B.S.E. in chemical engineering from Princeton University, and his M.D., magna cum laude, from the Harvard Medical School, and received the Robinson Award for Surgery. He earned his Ph.D. in biochemical engineering/biotechnology from the Massachusetts Institute of Technology, where he was named a

Hugh Hampton Young fellow. A practicing sports medicine and shoulder surgeon, Dr. Laurencin has been named to America's Top Doctors for over 15 years. He is a fellow of the American Academy of Orthopaedic Surgeons, a fellow of the American Orthopaedic Association, a fellow of the American College of Surgeons, and a member of the American Surgical Association. He received the Nicolas Andry Award, the highest honor of the Association of Bone and Joint Surgeons. Dr. Laurencin served as dean of the medical school and vice president for health affairs at the University of Connecticut. Dr. Laurencin is a pioneer of the new field of regenerative engineering. He is an expert in biomaterials science, stem cell technology, and nanotechnology and was named one of the 100 Engineers of the Modern Era by the American Institute of Chemical Engineers, and received the Founder's Award from the Society for Biomaterials. He received the NIH Director's Pioneer Award, NIH's highest and most prestigious research award, for his new field of regenerative engineering and the National Science Foundation's Emerging Frontiers in Research and Innovation Grant Award. Dr. Laurencin is the editor-in-chief of *Regenerative Engineering and Translational Medicine*, published by Springer Nature, and is the founder of the Regenerative Engineering Society. He is a fellow of the American Chemical Society, the American Institute of Chemical Engineers, the Biomedical Engineering Society, the Materials Research Society, and the American Association for the Advancement of Science (AAAS). The AAAS awarded Dr. Laurencin the Philip Hauge Abelson Prize given "for signal contributions to the advancement of science in the United States." Dr. Laurencin is active in mentoring, especially for underrepresented minority students. He received the AAAS Mentor Award, the Beckman Award for Mentoring, and the Presidential Award for Excellence in Science, Math and Engineering Mentoring in ceremonies at the White House. The Society for Biomaterials established the Cato T. Laurencin, M.D., Ph.D. Travel Fellowship in his honor, awarded to underrepresented minority students pursuing research. Dr. Laurencin is also active in addressing health disparities. Dr. Laurencin completed the program in African American Studies at Princeton University. He is a core faculty member of the Africana Studies Institute at the University of Connecticut, and is editor-in-chief of the *Journal of Racial and Ethnic Health Disparities*, published by Springer Nature. He co-founded the W. Montague Cobb/NMA Health Institute, dedicated to addressing health disparities, and served as its founding chair. The W. Montague Cobb/NMA Health Institute and the National Medical Association established the Cato T. Laurencin Lifetime Research Achievement Award, given during the opening ceremonies of the National Medical Association Meeting. Dr. Laurencin is an elected member of the National Academy of Medicine, an elected member of the National Academy of Engineering, and an elected member of the American Academy of Arts and Sciences. Active internationally, he is an elected fellow of the Indian National Academy of Sciences, the Indian National Academy of Engineering, the African Academy of Sciences, and the World Academy of Sciences, and is an academician of the Chinese Academy of Engineering.

Cora Bagley Marrett is professor emerita of sociology at the University of Wisconsin–Madison. She has held posts at the University of North Carolina, Chapel Hill; Western Michigan University; the University of Wisconsin System; and the University of Massachusetts Amherst. At UMass she was provost and vice chancellor for academic affairs. For 11 years she served as an administrator at the National Science Foundation (NSF), initially overseeing activities associated with the social and behavioral sciences and later, those centered on education and human resources. In her final years, she held the second ranking post at NSF: deputy director. She was appointed to that position by President Barack Obama and confirmed by the U.S. Senate. Over her career, she has served on governing or advisory boards with the Social Science Research Council; the Russell Sage Foundation; the National Academies of Sciences, Engineering and Medicine; and the Office of Naval Research, among others. At the request of President Jimmy Carter, she was a member of the body that examined the nuclear power incident in Pennsylvania: the Commission on the Accident at Three Mile Island. She holds honorary degrees from her undergraduate alma mater, Virginia Union University; the institution of her doctorate, the University of Wisconsin–Madison; and Wake Forest University.

Ebony O. McGee is an associate professor of diversity and STEM education at Vanderbilt University's Peabody College. She investigates what it means to be racially marginalized while minoritized in the context of learning and achieving in STEM higher education and in the STEM professions. In particular, Dr. McGee studies the racialized experiences and racial stereotypes that adversely affect the education and career trajectories of underrepresented groups of color. This involves exploring the social, material, and health costs of academic achievement and problematizing traditional forms of success in higher education, with an unapologetic focus on Black folk in these places and spaces. Her National Science Foundation

(NSF) CAREER grant investigates how marginalization undercuts success in STEM through psychological stress, interrupted STEM career trajectories, impostor phenomenon, and other debilitating race-related trauma for Black, Indigenous, and Latinx doctoral students. Education is her second career; Dr. McGee left a career in electrical engineering to earn a Ph.D. in mathematics education from the University of Illinois Chicago, a Spencer Postdoctoral Fellowship at the University of Chicago, and a National Science Foundation Postdoctoral Fellowship at Northwestern University. With funding from six NSF grants, she cofounded the Explorations in Diversifying Engineering Faculty Initiative, or EDEFI (pronounced "edify"). She also co-founded the Institute in Critical Quantitative and Mixed Methodologies Training for Underrepresented Scholars (ICQCM), which seeks to be a "go-to" institute for the development of quantitative and mixed-methods skill sets that challenge simplistic quantifications of race and marginalization. ICQCM was founded with support from the National Science Foundation, the Spencer Foundation, and the W. T. Grant Foundation. She is the lead editor of the recently published book *Diversifying STEM: Multidisciplinary Perspectives on Race and Gender* (2019), which offers scholarship that includes race, culture, and social stratification; racial justice and identity; racial socialization processes; and race and gender intersectionality in STEM. Dr. McGee's research has been featured in prominent media outlets, including *The Atlantic*, *Diverse Issues in Higher Education*, *The Chronicle of Higher Education*, NPR's *Codeswitch*, *The Hechinger Report*, *Christian Science Monitor*, *Huffington Post*, *U.S. News & World Report*, *Inside Higher Education*, *Tennessean*, and *The UK Voice Online*.

Valerie Montgomery Rice is the sixth president of Morehouse School of Medicine (MSM) and the first woman to lead the freestanding medical institution, where she serves as both the president and CEO. A renowned infertility specialist and researcher, she most recently served as dean and executive vice president of MSM, where she has served since 2011.

Prior to joining MSM, Dr. Montgomery Rice held faculty positions and leadership roles at various health centers, including academic health centers. Most notably, she was the founding director of the Center for Women's Health Research at Meharry Medical College, one of the nation's first research centers devoted to studying diseases that disproportionately impact women of color.

Dedicated to the creation and advancement of health equity, Dr. Montgomery Rice lends her vast experience and talents to programs that enhance pipeline opportunities for academically diverse learners, diversifies the physician and scientific workforce, and fosters equity in health-care access and health outcomes. To this end, she holds memberships in various organizations and participates on a number of boards, such as the following: member, National Academy of Medicine, the Association of American Medical Colleges Council of Deans, and the Horatio Alger Association and board of directors for the Metro Atlanta Chamber, Kaiser Permanente School of Medicine, the Nemours Foundation, UnitedHealth Group, Westside Future Fund, Josiah Macy Jr. Foundation, Headspace, Wellpath, and CARE.

Dr. Montgomery Rice has received numerous accolades and honors. She was named to the Horatio Alger Association of Distinguished Americans and received the 2017 Horatio Alger Award. For three consecutive years (2016–2018) *Georgia Trend* magazine selected her as one of the 100 Most Influential Georgians. Other honors include the following: the Dean Griffin Community Service Award from the Georgia Institute of Technology, Girls Inc. 2019 Smart Award, National Medical Association OB/GYN 2019 Legend of the Section Award, Turknett Leadership Character Award (2018), Visions of Excellence Award, Atlanta Business League (2018), Links Incorporated Co-Founders Award (2018), Trumpet Vanguard Award (2015), Dorothy I. Height Crystal Stair Award (2014), National Coalition of 100 Black Women—Women of Impact (2014), YWCA—Women of Achievement of Atlanta (2014) and Nashville (2007), American Medical Women's Association Elizabeth Blackwell Medal (2011), and Working Mother Media Multicultural Women's Legacy Award (2011).

A Georgia native, Dr. Montgomery Rice holds a bachelor's degree in chemistry from the Georgia Institute of Technology, a medical degree from Harvard Medical School, an honorary degree from the University of Massachusetts Medical School and a doctor of humane letters honorary degree from Rush University. All reflect her lifetime commitment to education, service, and the advancement of health equity. She completed her residency in obstetrics and gynecology at Emory University School of Medicine and her fellowship in reproductive endocrinology and infertility at Hutzel Hospital.

J. Nwando Olayiwola is the chief health equity officer and senior vice president for Humana. She is responsible for creating and implementing a strategy to achieve health equity across all lines of business, including care delivery, giving all communities and groups of people a fair and just opportunity to be as healthy as possible. Dr. Olayiwola leads cross-functional efforts for the organization's journey toward more equitable care.

A longtime advocate for underserved communities, Dr. Olayiwola brings more than 20 years of experience in clinical, community, and academic medicine, health technology leadership, public health, and domestic and international health systems redesign to Humana. Her October 2020 Tedx Talk is a clarion call for health equity.

Prior to joining Humana, Dr. Olayiwola was the chair and professor in the Department of Family and Community Medicine at the Ohio State University (OSU) College of Medicine, where she was also the founding director of the Center for Primary Care Innovation and Transformation and co-chair of the OSU Wexner Medical Center's Anti-Racism Action Plan. She previously served as chief clinical transformation officer for RubiconMD, director of the University of California, San Francisco, Center for Excellence in Primary Care, and chief medical officer of Community Health Center, Inc., Connecticut's largest Federally Qualified Health Center system. She continues to practice as a board-certified family physician, serving a largely medically underserved patient population.

Dr. Olayiwola was a Commonwealth Fund/Harvard University fellow in Minority Health Policy at Harvard Medical School from 2004 to 2005. During this fellowship and leadership training, she received her master's degree in public health with a concentration in health policy from the Harvard School of Public Health. She obtained her undergraduate degree in Human Nutrition/Pre-Medicine at the Ohio State University and her medical degree from the Ohio State University/Cleveland Clinic Foundation. She completed her residency training in family medicine at Columbia University/New York Presbyterian Hospital, where she was a chief resident. She is the recipient of numerous awards, including Family Physicians Who Are Changing Our World by the Family Medicine Education Consortium and the Woman of the Year Award by the American Telemedicine Association. Dr. Olayiwola is married and has two school-aged children.

Sudip Parikh became the 19th chief executive officer of the American Association for the Advancement of Science (AAAS) and executive publisher of the Science family of journals in January 2020. Dr. Parikh has spent two decades at the nexus of science, policy, and business.

Immediately prior to joining AAAS, Dr. Parikh was senior vice president and managing director at DIA Global, a neutral, multidisciplinary organization bringing together regulators, industry, academia, patients, and other stakeholders interested in health-care product development. He led strategy in the Americas and oversaw Defense Intelligence Agency programs that catalyzed progress globally toward novel regulatory frameworks for advanced therapies not amenable to existing regulations.

An active member of the scientific advocacy community, Dr. Parikh serves as a board member and officer for several impactful organizations, including Research!America, Friends of Cancer Research, and ACT for the National Institutes of Health (NIH). He has received multiple public service awards, including recognition from the American Association of Immunologists, the National AIDS Alliance, the Coalition for Health Services Research, and the Juvenile Diabetes Research Foundation.

Dr. Parikh is committed to early STEM education and, as a parent of three energetic young children, he prioritizes volunteering as a mentor for Science Olympiad teams at two elementary schools.

Early in his career, he was a presidential management intern at the NIH. He was awarded a National Science Foundation Graduate Research Fellowship while earning his Ph.D. in macromolecular structure and chemistry from the Scripps Research Institute in La Jolla, California. There, he used structural biology and biochemistry techniques to probe the mechanisms of DNA repair enzymes bound to DNA. The son of Indian immigrants who worked in the textile and furniture manufacturing plants of North Carolina, Dr. Parikh completed undergraduate studies at the University of North Carolina at Chapel Hill, first as a journalism major before switching into materials science.

Keivan Stassun is the Stevenson Professor of Physics & Astronomy, director of the Vanderbilt Initiative in Data-intensive Astrophysics (VIDA), and director of the Frist Center for Autism and Innovation at Vanderbilt University. After earning A.B. degrees in physics and astronomy from the University of California, Berkeley, and a Ph.D. in astrophysics from the University of Wisconsin, Dr. Stassun was a NASA Hubble postdoctoral fellow before joining the Vanderbilt faculty in 2003. A recipient of a CAREER award from the National Science Foundation (NSF) and a Cottrell Scholar Award from the Research Corporation for Science Advancement, his research on stars and exoplanets has appeared in more than 400 peer-reviewed journal articles. He is a co-investigator for the NASA Transiting Exoplanet Survey Satellite (TESS) mission and chairs the executive committee of the Sloan Digital Sky Survey. From 2004 to 2015, he served as founding director of the Fisk-Vanderbilt Master's-to-Ph.D.

Bridge Program, which has become one of the nation's top producers of Ph.D.'s to underrepresented minorities in the physical sciences. He has served on the federal Astronomy and Astrophysics Advisory Committee, the NSF Committee for Equal Opportunity in Science and Engineering, is a recipient of the American Physical Society's Nicholson Medal for Human Outreach, and is an elected fellow of the American Physical Society, American Astronomical Society, and American Association for the Advancement of Science (AAAS). He has served as an expert witness to the U.S. House of Representatives Committee on Science and Technology. For the past 10 years, Dr. Stassun has served as founding director of the Vanderbilt Initiative in Data-intensive Astrophysics. In 2017, he launched the Center for Autism and Innovation, focused on advancing science and engineering through the engagement and advancement of individuals with autism. The center has become permanently endowed by a $10 million gift from Frist Family Foundation. Most recently, he was selected for a $1 million HHMI Professor award, was named Mentor of the Year by the AAAS, was honored by the White House with a Presidential Award for Excellence in Science and Engineering Mentoring, and has been appointed to the National Academies' Decadal Steering Committee for Astronomy and Astrophysics.

Altha J. Stewart is senior associate dean for community health engagement and associate professor in psychiatry at the University of Tennessee Health Science Center (UTHSC) in Memphis, Tennessee. She also serves as director for the Division of Public and Community Psychiatry and director for the Center for Health in Justice Involved Youth in the Department of Psychiatry, where she manages community-based programs serving children impacted by trauma and mental illness and their families. Prior to joining the UTHSC College of Medicine faculty, she served as executive director of Memphis' federally funded System of Care Program for children with serious emotional disorders and their families. Dr. Stewart is the former executive director of the Detroit-Wayne County Community Mental Health Agency, one of the largest public mental health systems in the United States. She served as deputy commissioner and later interim commissioner of the former New York City Department of Mental Health, and CEO/executive director in other large public health and mental health systems in New York and Pennsylvania, overseeing the management and development of programs for persons with mental illness, substance use disorders, and justice system involvement. Dr. Stewart received her medical degree from Temple University Medical School, completing her psychiatric residency at what is now Drexel University. In 2017, she was elected the 145th president of the American Psychiatric Association, the first African American elected to this position in the 175-year history of the organization. She is also past president of the Black Psychiatrists of America, the Association of Women Psychiatrists, and the American Psychiatric Foundation. She has received numerous awards and honors, including visiting professorships at the Massachusetts General Hospital, University of Maryland, and University of California, Davis; honorary membership in the South African Society of Psychiatrists; honorary degrees from Regis College and Christian Brothers University; the National Alliance on Mental Illness (NAMI) Exemplary Psychiatrist Awards (2002 and 2020); and the American Psychological Association's (APA) Solomon Carter Fuller and Alexandra Symonds Awards.

Mike Summer received his A.A. degree in chemistry from St. Petersburg Junior College (1978), B.S. in chemistry from the University of West Florida (1980), Ph.D. in Bioinorganic Chemistry from Emory University (1984), and was a postdoctoral fellow at the National Institutes of Health (NIH) (1984–1987) before joining the faculty at the University of Maryland, Baltimore County (1987–present). In 1994 he was appointed as an investigator with the Howard Hughes Medical Institute, and in 2016 he was elected to the National Academy of Sciences. He was the recipient of two NIH MERIT Awards for studies of HIV structural biology. Currently, Dr. Summers is an associate editor for the *Proceedings of the National Academy of Sciences* and the *Journal of Molecular Biology*, and is a member of the editorial advisory board of the *Journal of Biomolecular NMR*. Dr. Summers' research focuses on NMR studies of proteins, RNA, and macromolecular interactions associated with HIV-1 genome packaging and virus assembly. His laboratory typically includes large numbers of students from diverse backgrounds. He has mentored more than 300 undergraduates in his lab. He has also led efforts to develop programs for retaining minority students in the sciences. He directs an NIH-funded diversity program that includes more than 100 enrolled underrepresented minority Ph.D. students. Dr. Summers is a recipient of the Ruth Kirstein Award of the American Society of Biochemistry and Molecular Biology; the Carl Branden Award of the Protein Society; the Emily M. Gray Mentoring Award of the Biophysical Society; the American Society for Biochemistry and Molecular Biology Award for Exemplary Contributions to Education; the Mentor Award of the American Association for the Advancement of Science; the American Society for Microbiology Hinton

Award for Mentoring; and the White House Presidential Award for Science, Mathematics, and Engineering Mentoring.

Laurie Zephyrin is vice president of advancing health equity at the Commonwealth Fund. Previously, she was vice president of delivery system reform. Her work at the Fund has included advancing health equity in delivery systems and health policy, promoting high-quality, comprehensive primary health care, and promoting equity-centered care for birthing people throughout the life-course. She combines her experience as a clinician, health policy maker, and health systems innovator to her role at the Commonwealth Fund to drive delivery system change. Dr. Zephyrin has extensive experience leading the vision, design, and delivery of innovative health-care models across national health systems. She was the first national director of the Reproductive Health Program at the Department of Veterans Affairs (VA), spearheading the strategic vision and leading systems change and policy to improve the health of women veterans nationwide; she served as acting assistant deputy under secretary for health for community care, and later, as acting deputy under secretary for health for community care. While directing the VA's Community Care program, Dr. Zephyrin spearheaded efforts to implement legislation, develop internal governance structures, and address patient outcomes through systemwide transformation of care delivery. As part of the leadership team, she also represented the VA before Congress and other internal and external stakeholders. Her perspective and experience as a systems thinker and a leader provides refreshing insight on health-care delivery and advancing health equity. She has written articles and has been featured in various publications, was named a White House fellow, Young Global Leader, Robert Wood Johnson Clinical Scholar, and Aspen Health Innovator fellow. Dr. Zephyrin earned her M.D. from the New York University School of Medicine, M.B.A. and M.P.H. from Johns Hopkins University, and B.S. in biomedical sciences from the City College of New York. She is a board-certified obstetrician and gynecologist and completed her residency training at Harvard's Integrated Residency Program at Brigham and Women's Hospital and Massachusetts General Hospital.

PLANNING COMMITTEE

Evelynn Hammonds (*Co-Chair*) is a member of the faculty in the Faculty of Arts and Sciences at Harvard University. She was the first senior vice provost for faculty development and diversity at Harvard (2005–2008). From

2008 to 2013, she served as dean of Harvard College. She holds honorary degrees from Spelman College and Bates College. Professor Hammonds is the director of the Project on Race & Gender in Science & Medicine at the Hutchins Center for African and African American Research at Harvard. Prof. Hammonds earned a Ph.D. in the history of science from Harvard University, an S.M. in physics from the Massachusetts Institute of Technology (MIT), a B.E.E. in electrical engineering from the Georgia Institute of Technology, and a B.S. in physics from Spelman College. In 2010 she was appointed to President Barack Obama's Board of Advisers on Historically Black Colleges and Universities and in 2014 to the President's Commission on Excellence in Higher Education for African Americans. She has published articles on the history of disease, race, and science, African American feminism, African American women and the epidemic of HIV/AIDS, and analyses of gender and race in science and medicine. Prof. Hammonds' current research focuses on diversity in science, technology, engineering, and mathematics (STEM) fields; the intersection of scientific, medical, and socio-political concepts of race in the United States; and genetics and society. She served two terms on the Committee on Equal Opportunity in Science and Engineering (CEOSE), the congressionally mandated oversight committee of the National Science Foundation (NSF). Prof. Hammonds was appointed to the Committee on Women in Science, Engineering, and Medicine (CWSEM) of the National Academies in 2017. She was elected to the National Academy of Medicine (NAM) in 2018.

Shirley Malcom (*Co-Chair*) is senior advisor and director of SEA Change, an institutional transformation initiative, at the American Association for the Advancement of Science (AAAS). In her more than 40-year tenure at the AAAS, she has worked to improve the quality and increase access to education and careers in science, technology, engineering, mathematics, and medicine (STEMM) for all women, BIPOC men (Black, Indigenous and People of Color), persons with disabilities and other marginalized groups, as well as to enhance public science literacy.

Dr. Malcom is a trustee of Caltech and regent of Morgan State University, an HBCU (Historically Black College and University). She is a former member of the National Science Board, the policy-making body of the U.S. National Science Foundation, and served on President Clinton's Committee of Advisors on Science and Technology. She is a native of Birmingham, Alabama, and received her Ph.D. in ecology from the Pennsylvania State University, master's in zoology from the University of California, Los

Angeles (UCLA), and bachelor's with distinction in zoology from the University of Washington. She has been recognized for her work and service by all of these institutions, being the recipient of the Distinguished Alumni Award from the Pennsylvania State University (2001), the UCLA Medal (2015), and Alumna Summa Laude Dignata of the University of Washington (1998). She is an elected fellow of the AAAS and a member of the American Academy of Arts and Sciences. In addition, she holds 17 honorary degrees.

Dr. Malcom is a former high school science teacher and university faculty member. She serves on the boards of the Heinz Endowments, Public Agenda, and Digital Promise Global. She also chairs the board of NMSI, the National Math and Science Initiative. In 2003, Dr. Malcom received the Public Welfare Medal of the U.S. National Academy of Sciences, the highest award given by the Academy.

Vivian Pinn (*Co-Chair*) was the first full-time director of the National Institutes of Health (NIH) Office of Research on Women's Health, an appointment she held since 1991 and as NIH associate director for research on Women's Health since 1994 prior to her retirement in August 2011. Since her retirement, she has been named as a senior scientist emerita at the NIH Fogarty International Center. Dr. Pinn came to NIH from Howard University College of Medicine in Washington, D.C., where she had been professor and chair of the Department of Pathology from 1982 until 1991. Dr. Pinn had previously held teaching appointments at Harvard Medical School and Tufts University, where she was also assistant dean for student affairs. A special tribute by Senator Olympia Snowe on Dr. Pinn's retirement was published in the Congressional Record in November 2011, commending her contributions during her NIH tenure. The Association of American Medical Colleges awarded her a Special Recognition Award for exceptional leadership over a 40-year career. She has received numerous honors and recognitions, and is a fellow of the American Academy of Arts and Sciences and was elected to the National Academy of Medicine (formerly the Institute of Medicine) in 1995. A graduate and Alumna Achievement Award recipient as well as former Trustee of Wellesley College, she earned her M.D. from the University of Virginia School of Medicine, the only woman or minority in her class. She completed her postgraduate training in pathology at the Massachusetts General Hospital. Dr. Pinn has received 17 honorary degrees of science, law, and medicine, and the University of Virginia School of Medicine has named one of its four advisory medical student colleges as

"The Pinn College" in her honor. Tufts University School of Medicine in 2011 announced "The Vivian W. Pinn Office of Student Affairs," named for her at the time her former medical students dedicated a scholarship in her name. She has held leadership positions in many professional organizations, including president of the National Medical Association (NMA) and is currently chair of the NMA Past Presidents Council. Dr. Pinn currently serves on the Board of Trustees/Advisors of Thomas Jefferson University and Tufts University School of Medicine. She was recently elected to Modern Healthcare's Hall of Fame, the first African American woman to be so honored, and received the Outstanding Woman Leader in Healthcare Award from the University of Michigan. Dr. Pinn also holds the position of professor at the Institute for Advanced Discovery and Innovation at the University of South Florida.

Kevin Cokley's research can be broadly categorized in the area of African American psychology, with a focus on racial and ethnic identity development, academic motivation, and academic achievement. A theme of much of his research is understanding the psychological and environmental factors that impact African American student achievement. Dr. Cokley's research and scholarship have led him to challenge the notion that African American students are anti-intellectual, and to critically reexamine the impact of racial and ethnic identity and gender on academic achievement. Recently he has started exploring the impostor phenomenon and its relationship to mental health and academic outcomes among ethnic minority students.

Dr. Cokley's publications have appeared in professional journals such as the *Journal of Counseling Psychology*, *Journal of Black Psychology*, *Cultural Diversity and Ethnic Minority Psychology*, *Individual Differences and Personality*, *Measurement and Evaluation in Counseling and Development*, the *Journal of Multicultural Counseling and Development*, *Educational and Psychological Measurement*, and the *Harvard Educational Review*.

He has a joint appointment in the College of Education's Department of Educational Psychology and the College of Liberal Arts' Department of African and African Diaspora Studies. He is the past editor-in-chief of the *Journal of Black Psychology* and the director of the Institute for Urban Policy Research & Analysis.

Dr. Cokley has written several op-eds in major media outlets, including the *St. Louis Post Dispatch*, *Dallas Morning News*, *San Antonio Express*, *The American Prospect*, *The Huffington Post*, *The Conversation*, and *The Hill* on topics such as Blacks rational mistrust of police, police shootings of Blacks, the aftermath of Ferguson, the use of school vouchers, racial disparities in school discipline, and Black students graduation rates.

Michellene Davis is a trailblazing leader and passionate voice for equity. A trial attorney by training, she spent her earliest years in public service representing disenfranchised members of the most vulnerable populations. An effective advocate and researcher, she became the first African American to serve as chief policy counsel within the New Jersey Governor's Office.

Prior to making history in the Governor's Office, Ms. Davis broke barriers in the New Jersey Department of the Treasury where, as the first African American woman state treasurer, she created the Treasury's first Office of Supplier Diversity and Division of Minority and Women-Owned Businesses in order to ensure equal access to revenue-generating opportunities for women and minority-owned businesses.

Before being appointed acting state treasurer, Ms. Davis was the youngest executive director and CEO of the New Jersey Lottery, where she generated record-setting revenue numbers. As a result of her financial achievements, the state of New Jersey was able to increase its General Fund contribution to education and state-run veterans homes. She was also the first woman and first person of color to rise to the executive vice president level at one of the largest health-care systems in the country.

An internationally requested speaker, she is an inspiring orator with a natural ability to connect and communicate while simultaneously challenging audiences. Her talents are surpassed only by her personal story. Beyond being a woman of numerous career "firsts," she has persevered through personal losses and adversity and continued to excel.

Ms. Davis has received national recognition for her professional accomplishments. In 2016, she received the Evangelina Menendez Trailblazer Award from U.S. Senator Robert Menendez, and she was also the recipient of the Corporate Sector Award from the New Jersey Women Lawyers Association. Previously, she was named the 2015 LUPE Amiga of the Year, the 2014 Business Advocate of the Year by the Statewide Hispanic Chamber of Commerce, and she was selected as one of *The Network Journal*'s 2014 Top 25 Most Influential Black Women in Business.

Ms. Davis is also active in her civic community. She serves as a member of the Board of Governors of Rowan University/Rutgers – Camden; a member of the New Jersey Performing Arts Center Women's Board; a member of the Board of Directors of the Caucus Educational Trust; a member of the Board of Executive Women of New Jersey (EWNJ); and a trustee of the

New Jersey Women Lawyers Association and the New Jersey Legislative Black Caucus Foundation.

Ms. Davis began her legal career as a trial litigator. She is an honors graduate of Seton Hall University, and she holds a juris doctorate from Seton Hall School of Law.

Garth Graham is a leading authority on social determinants of health. President of the Aetna Foundation and vice president of Community Health for Aetna, Inc., he is also a cardiologist and public health expert. Dr. Graham oversees the community health initiatives for the Aetna Foundation and Aetna, Inc., bringing his experience as a former deputy assistant secretary at the U.S. Department of Health and Human Services under the Obama and Bush administrations, where he also ran the Office of Minority Health. He directed the development of the federal government's first National Health Disparities Plan released under the Obama administration. Dr. Graham has been a contributor to *The Hill*, the *Chicago Tribune*, *Fortune*, *Quartz*, *Health Affairs*, and *Ebony*, and has been featured in *Essence*, *CNN*, and *The New York Times*, among others. His original research has been published in the *Journal of the American Medical Association*, *American Journal of Public Health*, *Health Affairs*, and other publications. Along with his role at the Aetna Foundation, Dr. Graham is a clinical associate professor of medicine at the University of Connecticut. Prior to joining the Foundation, in his role as the assistant dean for health policy at the University of Florida School of Medicine, he led several research initiatives looking at how to improve outcomes and readmission rates in cardiac patients in underserved populations. He contributes to several boards, including being named by the president to the U.S. Federal Coordinating Council on Comparative Effectiveness Research, the Institute of Medicine Board on Population Health, the American Heart Association/American Stroke Associational National Quality Oversight Committee, the American College of Cardiology/American Heart Association Task Force on Clinical Data Standards, and many others. Dr. Graham holds a medical degree from Yale School of Medicine, a master's in public health from Yale School of Public Health, and a bachelor of science in biology from Florida International University in Miami. He completed clinical training in cardiology and interventional cardiology at Massachusetts General Hospital and Johns Hopkins. He holds three board certifications: internal medicine, cardiology, and interventional cardiology.

Thomas A. Vance is a counseling psychologist, scholar, and researcher with over a decade of clinical experience, specializing in interdisciplinary psychology, collaborating with unrepresented communities in using their voice through necessary skills training. He currently serves as the director of implementation social services at the Boys and Girls Clubs of America (BGCA), where he is the lead social services expert, overseeing youth outreach and intervention programs around trauma-informed practices and safety and planning. Dr. Vance is also a visiting research scholar at the Schools for Public Engagement at the New School in New York City and the clinical director of his private practice, AdVance Perspectives, providing therapeutic care in Atlanta, Georgia. Dr. Vance utilizes evidence-based therapies to assist clients manage anxiety, mood disorders, behavioral symptoms, as well as sexual/gender concerns. As every client's background is unique, Dr. Vance believes in utilizing a social justice, intersectional, and multicultural framework to recognize the importance of one's identities in psychological development.

Prior to his time at the BGCA, Dr. Vance completed his teaching postdoctoral psychology fellowship at the New School for Social Research. Dr. Vance also completed his clinical and research postdoctoral fellowship at Columbia University Irving Medical Center (CUIMC), working within the Columbia Gender Identity Program. He received his doctorate in counseling psychology from the University of Akron in 2018. Amidst other commitments, Dr. Vance serves as a member of the Presidential Task Force on Advancing Social and Emotional Development of Black Boys through Research, Advocacy, and Community Engagement, as well as the co-chair of the American Psychological Association (APA), Division 17, and Diversity Committee member of APA, Division 53.

Dr. Vance's professional experiences have centered on uplifting social justice efforts with scientific evidence, while also ensuring scientific advancements are analyzed with multicultural considerations. His expertise lies in multivariate identity development, extensively working with individuals from marginalized backgrounds. His clinical and research-based practices examine the nature of stigmatized experiences, concentrating on their implications for psychosocial functioning—such as health and self-concept—and their intersections across axes of inequality.